Roberto Patarca-Montero, MD, PhD

Concise Encyclopedia
of Chronic Fatigue
Syndrome

*Pre-publication
REVIEWS,
COMMENTARIES,
EVALUATIONS . . .*

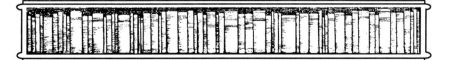

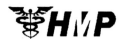

The Haworth Medical Press®
An Imprint of The Haworth Press, Inc.

Concise Encyclopedia
of Chronic Fatigue Syndrome

THE HAWORTH MEDICAL PRESS
Chronic Fatigue Syndrome, Fibromyalgia Syndrome, and Myalgic Encephalomyelitis

Roberto Patarca-Montero, MD, PhD
Senior Editor

Concise Encyclopedia of Chronic Fatigue Syndrome by Roberto Patarca-Montero

CFIDS, Fibromyalgia, and the Virus-Allergy Link: Hidden Viruses, Allergies, and Uncommon Fatigue/Pain Disorders by R. Bruce Duncan

Concise Encyclopedia of Chronic Fatigue Syndrome

Roberto Patarca-Montero, MD, PhD

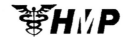

The Haworth Medical Press®
An Imprint of The Haworth Press, Inc.
New York • London • Oxford

Published by

The Haworth Medical Press®, an imprint of The Haworth Press, Inc., 10 Alice Street, Binghamton, NY 13904-1580

DISCLAIMER

Medicine is an ever-changing science. As new research and clinical experience broaden our knowledge, changes in treatment and drug therapy are required. While many suggestions for drug usages are made herein, the book is intended for educational purposes only, and the author, editor, and publisher do not accept liability in the event of negative consequences incurred as a result of information presented in this book. We do not claim that this information is necessarily accurate by the rigid, scientific standard applied for medical proof, and therefore make no warranty, expressed or implied, with respect to the material herein contained. Therefore the patient is urged to check the product information sheet included in the package of each drug he or she plans to administer to be certain the protocol followed is not in conflict with the manufacturer's inserts. When a discrepancy arises between these inserts and information in this book, the physician is encouraged to use his or her best professional judgement.

Cover design by Jennifer M. Gaska.

Library of Congress Cataloging-in-Publication Data

Patarca-Montero, Roberto.
    Concise encyclopedia of chronic fatigue syndrome / Roberto Patarca-Montero.
      p. ; cm.
    Includes bibliographical references and index.
    ISBN 0-7890-0922-6 (hard : alk. paper)—ISBN 0-7890-0923-4 (pbk. : alk. paper)
    1. Chronic fatigue syndrome—Encyclopedias. I. Title: Chronic fatigue syndrome. II. Title.
    [DNLM: 1. Fatigue Syndrome, Chronic—Encyclopedias—English. WB 13 P294c 2000]
RB150.F37 P38 2000
616'.0478'03—dc21

                                                 99-056033

CONTENTS

ABOUT THE AUTHOR

Roberto Patarca-Montero, MD, PhD, HCLD, is Assistant Professor of Medicine, Microbiology, and Immunology and also serves as Research Director of the E. M. Papper Laboratory of Clinical Immunology at the University of Miami School of Medicine. Previously, he was Assistant Professor of Pathology at the Dana-Farber Cancer Institute and Harvard Medical School in Boston. Dr. Patarca-Montero serves as Editor of *Critical Reviews in Oncogenesis* and the *Journal of Chronic Fatigue Syndrome.* He is also the author or co-author of more than 80 articles in journals or books. He is currently conducting research on immunotherapy of AIDS and chronic fatigue syndrome. Dr. Patarca-Montero is a member of the Board of Directors of the American Association for Chronic Fatigue Syndrome and the Acquired Non-HIV Immune Diseases Foundation.

Preface

Although much has been learned over the last decade about chronic fatigue syndrome (CFS), much remains to be learned about its causes, nosology, and treatment. Advances in cardiovascular medicine, endocrinology, epidemiology, immunology, infectious diseases, neurology, psychiatry, and psychology have served as the basis for the formulation of new lines of research and novel therapeutic interventions. Although old controversies as to what factors are more prominent in causation or perpetuation of CFS continue, they have not quenched progress in the field. The purpose of this *Concise Encyclopedia* is to summarize the knowledge gained and published mainly within the last three years. The text has been organized in such a way that the reader can easily access and become familiar with the highlights of the most relevant topics. A balanced view is presented in each category, and the lessons learned in related fatiguing disorders are also included. Evidence-based alternative medicine approaches for CFS are not included in this text since they are the subject of another publication by the same author. It is the hope of the author that this compendium will inspire more research into the field of CFS and that it will serve to educate and create greater awareness among health care professionals and the general public on this widespread and growing problem.

List of Abbreviations

ACTH	Adrenocorticotropin hormone
ADH	Antidiuretic hormone
ADP	Adenosine diphosphate
ANA	Antinuclear antibody
ATP	Adenosine triphosphate
BCAA	Branched-chain amino acids
BDV	Borna disease virus
CDC	Centers for Disease Control and Prevention
CDS	Cognitive Difficulty Scale
CFS	Chronic fatigue syndrome
CFSUM	Chronic fatigue symptom urinary marker
CID	Cellular immunodeficiency
CMV	Cytomegalovirus
CNS	Central nervous system
CRH	Corticotropin-releasing hormone
CS	Chemical sensitivity
CSF	Cerebrospinal fluid
DNA	Deoxyribonucleic acid
EBV	Epstein-Barr virus
ECP	Eosinophil cationic protein
EEG	Electroencephalograph
EPO	Erythropoietin
FIS	Fatigue Impact Scale
GH	Growth hormone
HLA-DQ3	Histocompatibility locus antigen DQ3
HPA	Hypothalamus-pituitary-adrenal axis
ICAM	Intercellular adhesion molecule
IFN	Interferon
IGF	Insulin-like growth factor
IL	Interleukin
LFA	Leucocyte functional antigen

MAO	Monoamine oxidase
MCS	Multiple chemical sensitivity syndrome
MMPI	Minnesota Multiphasic Personality Inventory
MRI	Magnetic resonance imaging
mRNA	Messenger ribonucleic acid
MS	Multiple sclerosis
NK	Natural killer cells
NO	Nitric oxide
PBMCs	Peripheral blood mononuclear cells
PCR	Polymerase chain reaction
PET	Positron emission tomography
PHA	Phytohemagglutinin
PKR	Protein kinase ribonucleic acid
PLS	Post-Lyme disease syndrome
PTSD	Post-traumatic stress disorder
PWA	Pokeweed mitogen
QOL	Quality of life
QUIN	Quinolinic acid
RAS	Reticular activating system
RAST	Radioallergosorbent test
REM	Rapid Eye Movement
RNA	Ribonucleic acid
RT-PCR	Reverse transcriptase-coupled polymerase chain reaction
SATET	Subanaerobic threshold exercise test
SBI	Silicone breast implant
SBS	Sick building syndrome
SCL	Symptom core list
SIADH	Syndrome of serum inappropriate anti-diuretic hormone
SLE	Systemic lupus erythematosus
SPECT	Single photon-emission computed tomography
TF	Transfer factor
TGF	Tumor growth factor
TNF	Tumor necrosis factor
UFC	Urinary free cortisol

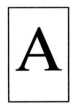

Acquired immunodeficiency syndrome (AIDS) and fatigue: Fatigue is a common and troubling symptom in patients with human immunodeficiency virus (HIV) infection and AIDS, and it results in significant disability with an adverse impact on activities of daily living and overall quality of life.[1-4] The etiology of HIV infection-associated fatigue remains complex and it is most likely multifactorial. Recognizable causes and correlates for which interventions can be beneficial include anemia, pain, infection/fever, hormonal or nutritional deficiencies, depression/anxiety, sleep disturbances, and excessive inactivity or rest.[1-4] It should also be noted that against a background of HIV infection-related fatigue, some forms of therapy such as that with interleukin-2 dramatically increase the experience of fatigue.[5] Poor sleep, daytime fatigue, and loss of cognitive ability exist during all stages of HIV infection, symptoms that worsen with disease progression. Data from several research groups support a role of somnogenic inflammation-related peptides whose levels are elevated in HIV infection, such as tumor necrosis factor-alpha. Although the literature is in conflict regarding an effect of HIV infection on growth hormone (GH) secretion, GH axis dysregulation and treatment with GH may be important in some complications of HIV infection, such as the wasting syndrome.[6] Fatigue declines significantly among responders to testosterone therapy in HIV seropositive men with clinical hypogonadism.[7,8] *See also* CYTOKINES, LOW CYSTEINE-GLUTATHIONE SYNDROME.

Age: *See* DEMOGRAPHICS.

Adrenocorticotropin hormone (ACTH): *See* NEUROENDOCRINOLOGY.

Akureyri disease: *See* ICELAND DISEASE.

Allergies: The elevated serum levels of eosinophil cationic protein (ECP) determined in one study suggest eosinophil activation.[1] In the same study, the prevalence of radioallergosorbent test (RAST) positivity to one or more allergens was 77 percent, while no control showed positive RAST. Twelve of the 14 CFS patients with increased ECP serum levels were RAST-positive. However, CFS RAST-positive patients had no significantly higher ECP serum levels than CFS RAST-negative patients, an observation that leaves open the question as to whether eosinophil activation has a pathogenetic role in CFS or whether a common immunologic background may exist for both atopy and CFS.

Although a higher prevalence of allergy[2,3] and delayed type hypersensitivity[4,5] can be detected in CFS patients, a trial with antihistamine treatment did not provide evidence of significant improvement,[6] and other studies[7] found no significant difference in the incidence of delayed type hypersensitivity and allergic responses among CFS patients. One group[8] found that while 30 percent of CFS patients had positive skin tests, an observation that suggests the potential for allergic rhinitis complaints, 46 percent had nonallergic rhinitis, an observation that, in turn, suggests that while atopy may coexist in some CFS subjects, it is unlikely to play a causal role. Another team[9] proposed that in at least a large subgroup of subjects with CFS with allergies, the concomitant influences of immune activation brought on by allergic inflammation in an individual with the appropriate psychologic profile may interact to produce the symptoms of CFS. This line of reasoning is underscored by a South African study[10] which suggested that food intolerance, in a genetically predisposed group of people, causes symptoms akin to both the major and minor criteria of CFS and that these individuals should be screened for such an allergy to avoid confusion. It may be possible that CFS and atopy share some common denominators, one of which may be the proposed Th2 (humoral immunity-oriented) cytokine predominant pattern in CFS. *See also* CYTOKINES, LYMPHOCYTES.

Amantadine: *See* MUSCLE PHYSIOLOGY.

Ankylosing spondylitis: *See* CONNECTIVE TISSUE AND RHEUMATOLOGIC DISORDERS.

Antidiuretic hormone (ADH)/Arginine vasopressin: A significant clinical overlap has been noted between chronic fatigue disorders and the syndrome of serum inappropriate antidiuretic hormone

(SIADH), which is characterized by lethargy and mental confusion, induction or exacerbation by viral illnesses, physical exertion, emotional stress and/or hypotension, and response to treatment with salt loading and glucocorticoids. Based on the latter observation, salt loading and/or direct inhibition of arginine vasopressin was proposed as a therapeutic approach in individuals with chronic fatigue disorders. *See* AUTONOMIC FUNCTION, BLOOD VOLUME.[1] One study[2] showed that, among CFS patients with evidence of autonomic dysfunction, a beneficial response to salt loading (1,200 mg of sodium chloride in a sustained-release formulation for three weeks) could be seen and those who did not respond had an abnormal renin-angiotensin-aldosterone system.

Anxiety disorders: *See* PSYCHOPATHOLOGY.

Apoptosis: Apoptosis, the process of programmed cell death, is regulated by several genes including *bax* and *bcl-2*. The bcl-2 protein forms a heterodimer with bax that inhibits apoptosis, whereas the bax-bax homodimer promotes it. A report[1] revealed increased expression of the apoptosis repressor ratio of bcl-2/bax in both CD4+ and CD8+ cells. However, recent evidence indicates that induction of apoptosis might be mediated in a dysregulated immune system, such as that present in CFS, by the upregulation of growth inhibitory cytokines and not the bcl-2 and bax pathways. In this respect, one group[2] found a larger apoptotic cell population in CFS individuals as compared to healthy controls. The increased apoptotic subpopulation in CFS individuals was associated with an abnormal cell arrest in the S phase and in the G2/M boundary of the cell cycle as compared to controls. In addition, CFS individuals exhibited enhanced mRNA and protein levels of the interferon (IFN)-induced protein kinase RNA (PKR) product, a mediator of apoptosis, as compared to healthy controls. In 50 percent of the CFS samples treated with 2-aminopurine (a potent inhibitor of PKR), the apoptotic population was reduced by more than 50 percent. PKR-mediated apoptosis may therefore contribute to the pathogenesis and the fatigue symptomatology associated with CFS. One research team[3] found that addition of a glyconutrient compound (dietary supplement that supplies the crucial eight monosaccharides required for synthesis of glycoproteins) to peripheral blood cells of CFS patients in vitro significantly decreased the percentage of apoptotic cells.

In contrast to the studies described above, one group[4] found no obvious difference in apoptosis in leukocyte cultures from CFS patients.

Atopy: *See* ALLERGIES.

Attention: *See* NEUROPSYCHOLOGY.

Attributions: *See* ILLNESS BELIEFS.

Autoantibodies: *See* AUTOIMMUNITY.

Autoimmunity: One research team[1] found that approximately 52 percent of sera from CFS patients react with nuclear envelope antigens. Some scra immunoprecipitated the nuclear envelope protein lamin B1, an observation which favors an autoimmune component in CFS.[2] Another report[3] documented a high frequency (83 percent) of autoantibodies to insoluble cellular antigens (vimentin and lamin B1) in CFS, a unique feature which might help to distinguish CFS from other rheumatic autoimmune diseases. The possible autoimmune etiology of CFS is further underscored by the significant association between CFS and the presence of histocompatibility locus antigen DQ3 (HLA-DQ3).[4]

Several studies have documented the presence in CFS patients of rheumatoid factor,[5-12] antinuclear antibodies,[3,5-7,9-14] antithyroid antibodies,[12,15,16] anti-smooth-muscle antibodies,[15] antigliadin, cold agglutinins, cryoglobulins, and false serological positivity for syphilis.[11,15] No circulating antimuscle and anti-central nervous system (CNS) antibodies were found in ten CFS patients[17] and one group[18] found no significant differences in the number of positive tests for autoantibodies in CFS patients.

One team[19] found that among children who chronically complain of nonspecific symptoms such as headache, fatigue, abdominal pain, and low grade fever, those who were antinuclear antibody (ANA) positive tended to have general fatigue and low grade fever, while gastrointestinal problems such as abdominal pain, diarrhea, and orthostatic dysregulation symptoms were commonly seen in ANA-negative patients. Children who were unable to go to school more than one day a week were seen significantly more among ANA-positive patients than among negative patients. Based on these observations, the authors concluded that autoimmunity may play a role in childhood chronic nonspecific symptoms and proposed a new disease entity: the autoimmune fatigue syndrome in children.

Autonomic function: Several studies have reported a close association between CFS and disturbances in the autonomic regulation of blood pressure and pulse, which are evident as neurally mediated hypotension or the postural tachycardia syndrome.[1-9] The latter two conditions can be induced by using tilt-table testing, which involves laying the patient horizontally on a table and then tilting the table upright to 70 degrees for 45 minutes while monitoring blood pressure and heart rate. Persons with neurally mediated hypotension or the postural tachycardia syndrome will develop lowered blood pressure and higher heart rate (palpitations) under these conditions, as well as other characteristic symptoms such as lightheadedness, weakness, visual dimming, or a slow response to verbal stimuli. The latter symptoms are relieved by resuming a supine posture. Many CFS patients show signs of abnormal vasovagal or vasodepressor responses to upright posture as evinced by their experience of lightheadedness or worsened fatigue when they stand for prolonged periods or when in warm places, such as in a hot shower. Autonomic impairment in CFS pediatric patients is suggested by depression of heart rate variability indices even when compared to children with syncope or controls: sympathovagal balance does not shift toward enhanced sympathetic modulation of heart rate with head-up tilt and there is blunting in the overall heart rate variability response with syncope during head-up tilt.[10]

In terms of the reasons for the presence of orthostatic intolerance and other symptoms of autonomic dysfunction, CFS is also associated with changes in neuroendocrine function, such as hypocortisolism (*see* NEUROENDOCRINOLOGY), and several reports have explored the links between neuroendocrine function disturbances, fatigue, and autonomic dysfunction. A study on the prevalence of fatigue assessed in a nonspecific pre-examination questionnaire by 431 patients, each subsequently diagnosed as having one of eight neurological or endocrine disorders, revealed that although fatigue commonly results from delayed orthostatic hypotension and all forms of hypocortisolism, it is less common in patients with acute orthostatic hypotension, both idiopathic and secondary to multiple system atrophy, which is more commonly present with lightheadedness or syncope.[11,12] The Addison type overtraining syndrome provides another example of a link between hypocortisolism, fatigue, and autonomic dysfunction. *See* OVERTRAINING.[13] During heavy endurance training or overreaching periods, a reduced adrenal responsiveness to ACTH is no longer compensated by an increased pituitary ACTH release, and the pituitary ACTH release also decreases with a concomitantly decreased intrinsic sympathetic activity and sensitivity of target organs to catecholamines. This is indicated by decreased catecholamine excretion during night rest, decreased beta-adrenoreceptor density, decreased beta-adrenoreceptor-mediated responses, and increased resting plasma norepinephrine levels and responses to exercise. These observations can explain persistent performance incompetence in affected athletes.[13] A study of vagal power during walking in CFS patients reported that in each of four periods of walking and in one of three periods of rest, CFS patients had significantly less vagal power than the control subjects despite there being no significant groupwise differences in mean heart rate, tidal volume, minute volume, respiratory rate, oxygen consumption, or total spectrum power. Furthermore, patients had a significant decline in resting vagal power after periods of walking. These results suggest a subtle abnormality in vagal activity to the heart in patients with the CFS and may explain, in part, their post-exertional symptom exacerbation.[14]

One study suggests that orthostatic intolerance and other symptoms of autonomic dysfunction in CFS may be explained by cardiovascular deconditioning, a postviral idiopathic autonomic neuropathy, or both.[3] *See* CARDIOVASCULAR DECONDITIONING. Besides impaired vasomotor tone, deconditioning, and autonomic neuropathy, hypovolemia may be a factor that could be influenced by hormonal or cytokine imbalances. *See* ANTIDIURETIC HORMONE (ADH)/ARGININE VASOPRESSIN, BLOOD VOLUME. Psychosomatic factors may also influence the occurrence of orthostatic dysregulation in young men as suggested by a study where the percentage classed in categories suggestive of emotional or psychological disturbance, according to the personality test, was 42.1 percent in those with orthostatic dysregulation and 8.9 percent in the controls.[15]

In contrast to the data discussed above, some groups argue that the findings of increased heart rate and higher low frequency power after tilting, which point to sympathetic overactivity and no parasympathetic abnormalities, provide no real explanation for the fatigue and intolerance to physical exertion in CFS patients.[16] Furthermore, several studies have failed to document an association between autonomic function impairment and CFS. One study of 19 CFS patients and 11 controls showed that autonomic function, as assessed by an analysis of heart rate variability during a two-stage tilt-table test while wearing a Holter monitor, does not differ in the baseline supine state, nor in response to upright tilt among CFS patients and healthy controls.[17] In the baseline supine position, high frequency (HF) power, low frequency (LF) power, and the ratio of low frequency power to high frequency power (LF/HF ratio) were similar. In both patient groups, upright tilt resulted in a similar decrease in HF power, increase in LF power, and increase in the LH/HF ratio.[17] Another report argued that many CFS patients examined by the tilt test had had orthostatic symptoms prior to the examination; that it is not certain that cardiovascular dysregulation is present in CFS patients without orthostatic symptoms; and that it is also not clear whether such a dysregulation would be the effect of physical inactivity or a manifestation of a subtle form of autonomic neuropathy.[18] One study reported that although higher heart rate and lower spectral indices of blood pressure variability while supine were found in CFS patients, analysis of RR-interval variability could not detect major alterations in autonomic function in CFS.[19] Another study documented the absence in CFS of denervation hypersensitivity of the sympathetic system, as assessed by a standardized supersensitivity test of pupil size (1.0 percent topical phenylephrine).[20]

Despite the negative associations described above, some interventions in cases of proven abnormal tilt test results have been beneficial. For instance, in a case comparison study with follow-up of eight weeks of a group of 78 CFS patients and 38 healthy controls,[6] patients with orthostatic hypotension by tilt test assessment at entry were offered therapy with sodium chloride (1,200 mg) in a sustained-release formulation for three weeks, prior to resubmission to the tilt-table testing, and clinical and laboratory evaluation. An abnormal response to upright tilt was observed in 22 of 78 patients with CFS. After sodium chloride therapy for eight weeks, tilt-table testing was repeated on the 22 patients with an abnormal response at baseline. Of these 22 patients, ten redeveloped orthostatic hypotension, while 11 did not show an abnormal response to the test and reported an improvement of CFS symptoms. However, those CFS patients who again developed an abnormal response to tilt test had a significantly reduced plasma renin activity (0.79 pmol/ml per h) compared with both healthy controls (1.29 pmol/ml per h) and those 11 CFS patients (1.0 pmol/ml per h) who improved after sodium chloride therapy.[6] Another therapeutic intervention involves the selective alpha-adrenergic agonist midrodrine, administration of a single dose of which before hemodialysis has been proven as an effective therapy for intradialytic hypotension where autonomic dysfunction is thought to play a significant role.[21] There is one report of successful head-up tilt-guided therapy.[22] Controlled therapeutic trials for CFS are underway.

B

Beta-2 microglobulin: Beta-2 microglobulin is a marker of immune activation and a marker for HIV-associated disease progression. Three studies found elevated levels of beta-2 microglobulin in patients with CFS[1-3] and one study found no difference.[4]

Blood volume: A high prevalence and frequent severity of low red blood cell mass was found among CFS patients, an observation that suggests that a reduction in oxygen-carrying power of the blood reaching the brain may contribute to CFS symptomatology.[1] Studies underway are assessing possible abnormalities in erythropoietin (EPO) production in CFS and the influence of cytokines such as tumor necrosis factor, which are known to inhibit EPO production[2] and whose serum levels are increased in a subset of CFS patients.[3]

Borna disease virus (BDV): Borna disease virus is a neurotropic, nonsegmented, negative-sense single-strand RNA virus. Natural infection with this virus has been reported to occur in horses and sheep. Recent epidemiological data suggest that BDV may be closely associated with neuropsychiatric disease (depression and schizophrenia) in humans. In Japanese patients with CFS, the prevalence of BDV infection is up to 34 percent. Furthermore, anti-BDV antibodies and BDV RNA were detected in a family cluster with CFS. These results suggest that BDV or a related agent may contribute to or initiate CFS, although the single etiologic role of BDV is unlikely.[1-3]

Brain injury and fatigue: In one study, patients with brain injury were found to experience significant levels of fatigue and the Fatigue Impact Scale (FIS) provided the most comprehensive examination of fatigue.[1] One proposal under investigation is that type I Chiari malformation or spinal cord compression by protrusion of cerebellar tonsils may underlie some cases of CFS.

Brain positron emission tomography (PET): *See* NEUROIMAGING.

Branched-chain amino acids (BCAA): *See* NUTRITION.

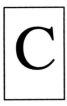

Cancer and fatigue: Higher incidences of non-Hodgkin's lymphoma and primary brain tumors, but not of breast or lung cancer, were noted in two northern Nevada counties (Washoe and Lyon) where outbreaks of a fatiguing illness, including cases of CFS, had been documented, compared to a southern Nevada county (Clark), where no such illness was reported.[1] The study concluded that a link between neoplasia and the fatiguing illness was premature and required further study.[1]

Cross-sectional studies suggest that fatigue in cancer patients is the result of a combination of physical and psychological causes.[2] For instance, women with breast cancer are at high risk for fatigue as a side effect of treatment with surgery, radiation, and chemotherapy, and the fatigue experience includes a physical component of decreased functional status, an affective component of emotional distress, and a cognitive component of difficulty concentrating.[3] Cancer patients, in general, typically experience fatigue while undergoing treatment for their diseases and oncologists' perceptions may not accurately reflect their patients' reported physical and psychosocial experiences.[4-12] In one study,[13] factors associated with greater fatigue severity included: female gender, presence of metastatic disease, and poorer performance status. In addition, the oldest patients were found to have less fatigue, as were patients with breast cancer, while patients with ovarian and lung cancer experienced greater fatigue. Patients on the arm of the anti-emetic trial in which emesis was better controlled showed significantly less increase in fatigue after receiving chemotherapy. Fatigue may also interfere with cancer therapy compliance and even limit the amount of treatment that a patient receives.[6]

In terms of after-treatment symptomatology, one group[14-16] reported that fatigue in disease-free post-radiotherapy cancer patients did not differ significantly from fatigue in the general population. However, for 34 percent of the patients, fatigue following treatment was worse than anticipated, 39 percent listed fatigue as one of the three symptoms causing them most distress, 26 percent of patients worried about their fatigue, and patients' overall quality of life was negatively related to fatigue. Fatigue in disease-free patients was significantly associated with gender, physical distress, pain rating, sleep quality, functional disability, psychological distress and depression, but not with medical (diagnosis, prognosis, co-morbidity) or treatment-related (target area, total radiation dose, fractionation) variables. The degree of fatigue, functional disability, and pain before radiotherapy were the best predictors of fatigue at nine-month follow-up. The significant associations between fatigue and both psychological and physical variables demonstrate the complex etiology of this symptom in patients and point out the necessity of a multidisciplinary approach for its treatment. Another study[17] found that fatigue in breast cancer survivors varies by type of cancer therapy.

An aerobic exercise program of precisely defined intensity, duration, and frequency can be prescribed as therapy for primary fatigue in cancer patients.[18] *See also* EXERCISE.

Cardiovascular deconditioning: A study[1] of 273 CFS patients provided evidence of physical and cardiovascular deconditioning (smaller left ventricular end systolic and diastolic dimensions, reduced left ventricular mass, smaller maximum and minimum diameter of the carotid artery, increased fat mass among males, and decreased serum albumin, phosphate, HDL-cholesterol, neutrophils, and thyroid-stimulating hormone). The authors suggested that in CFS patients a graded exercise program could lead to physical reconditioning and could increase their ability to perform physical activities. Another study[2] using measurements of heart rate, oxygen uptake, ventilation, and relative perceived exertion responses to incremental walking exercise up to volitional exhaustion in CFS subjects suggested that the limited exercise capacity in CFS subjects may be explained by deconditioning due to the sedentary lifestyle necessitated by the condition, coupled with an increased perception of exertion, potentially linked to psychological symptoms associated with CFS. *See also* EXERCISE.

Celiac disease: *See* GASTROINTESTINAL PATHOLOGY.

Chlorinated hydrocarbons: Environmental toxins have been studied as potential causes of CFS. A study of the potential relationships between chlorinated hydrocarbon contamination in human serum and red/white blood cell profiles, and an assessment of cellular response patterns to high and low serum organochlorine levels revealed that patients with unexplained and persistent fatigue had significantly higher levels of DDE (1,1-dichloro-2,2-bis(p-chlorophenyl) ethene) and different specific blood cell responses to organochlorines compared with controls. The red cell distribution width was elevated in the high DDE group and it was the most important discriminant parameter for differentiating between the high and low DDE groups.[1,2] Nonetheless, there is no clear association between CFS and chlorinated hydrocarbons.

Chronic fatigue syndrome (CFS), definition: Chronic fatigue syndrome is a disease entity of so far unknown etiopathogenesis without specific markers that presents with a complex array of symptoms in patients with diverse health histories. Fatigue is one of the most prominent features of CFS and one of the most common medical complaints in general. Patients with unexplained chronic pain and/or fatigue have been described for centuries in the medical literature, although the terms used to describe these symptom complexes have changed frequently. Neurasthenia dominated medical thinking at the turn of the century; the term "myalgic encephalomyelitis" was introduced in the United Kingdom in 1957 and in the mid-1980s, the term "chronic Epstein-Barr virus syndrome" emerged. Chronic Epstein-Barr virus syndrome was then converted to chronic fatigue syndrome and, by some, to "chronic fatigue immune dysfunction syndrome." The currently preferred term, albeit a misnomer, is chronic fatigue syndrome, a name which describes the prominent clinical features of the illness without any attempt to identify the cause, but has the endorsement of the United States Centers for Disease Control and Prevention (CDC) and several professional organizations. Related diseases include fibromyalgia, sick building syndrome, Gulf War syndrome, and multiple chemical sensitivity syndrome. Opinions on CFS range from nondisease via psychiatric disorder to a somatic disturbance. Nevertheless, CFS has emerged as a public health concern over the past decade in many countries and some court rulings have legitimized the diagnosis of CFS in some societal settings.

The diagnosis of CFS is based on clinical criteria and it is largely dependent upon ruling out other organic and psychologic causes of fatigue. CFS is defined by primary and secondary criteria that are, however, largely subjective. CFS includes cases of long-standing (six months or longer) fatigue that are not explained by an existing medical or psychiatric diagnosis and cause considerable disabilities in professional, social, and/or personal functioning (at least 50 percent reduction in baseline level). Other CFS criteria include: fever, painful adenopathy, muscle weakness, myalgia, headache, migratory arthralgia, neuropsychologic symptoms, and sleep disorder. Although several studies have validated these criteria, much controversy persists and attempts at formulating new criteria based on laboratory parameters are being undertaken. The working case definition of CFS in 1988 was an attempt to establish a uniform basis for the previously heterogeneous approaches to research of this severe and inexplicable state of fatigue. At the same time, researchers wished to narrow down a pathogenetically founded disease entity a priori by specifying precise disease criteria. The case definition has also been used to establish prevalence estimates using physician-based surveillance and random digit dial telephone surveys. Although the original 1988 definition was revised in 1994, the empirical data gathered in accordance with the CFS definition have failed to confirm the assumption that the disease entity is pathogenetically uniform.

The onset of CFS may be associated with preceding stressful events and multiple other precipitants. A study that divided CFS patients into two groups based on whether onset was sudden or gradual found that the rate of concurrent psychiatric disease was significantly greater in the CFS-gradual group relative to the CFS-sudden group. While both CFS groups showed a significant reduction in information processing ability relative to controls, impairment in memory was more severe in the CFS-sudden group. Some authors also make a distinction between an acute phase (up to one month after the first consultation), a subacute phase (until six months after the onset of the complaints and disabilities), and a chronic phase (from six months after the onset of the complaints and disabilities) of the disease. CFS evolves toward chronicity in an important number of cases.

Somatic pathogenetic hypotheses for CFS include persisting infections, intoxications, metabolic or immunologic disturbances, nervous system diseases, endocrine pathology, and psychosomatic influences. An infectious illness is not uniformly present at the onset and no single infectious agent has been found. Various components of the central nervous system appear to be involved in CFS, including the hypothalamic pituitary axes, pain-processing pathways, sleep-wake cycle, and autonomic nervous system. Many studies have provided evidence for abnormalities in immunological markers among individuals diagnosed with CFS. Nonetheless, a clear picture has not been achieved in any area of research because of the noticeable variability in the nature and magnitude of the findings reported by different groups. Moreover, little support has been garnered for an association between the laboratory abnormalities and the diverse physical and health status changes in the CFS population. For instance, some authors think that although a subset of CFS patients with immune system activation can be identified, serum markers of inflammation and immune activation are of limited diagnostic usefulness in the evaluation of patients with CFS and chronic fatigue because changes in their values may reflect an intercurrent, transient, common condition, such as an upper respiratory infection, or may be the result of an ongoing illness-associated process. On the other hand, other authors have found that CFS patients can be categorized based on immunological findings or that when patients are classified according to whether the disease started suddenly or gradually, immunological changes are apparent. It is also worth noting that although the degree of overlap between distributions of soluble immune mediators in CFS and controls has fueled criticism on the validity or clinical significance of immune abnormalities in CFS, the latter degree of overlap is not unique to CFS and is also present, for instance, in sepsis syndrome and HIV-1-associated disease, clinical entities where studies of immune abnormalities are providing insight into pathophysiology. The latter statement also applies to nonimmunological parameters in CFS.

Based on the discrepancies described above, some authors argue that the conceptual model of CFS needs to be changed from one determined by a single cause/agent to one in which dysfunction is the end stage of a multifactorial process. A study of author bias in literature citation in CFS reviews revealed that citation of literature is influenced by the author's discipline and nationality, a finding which is compatible with the lack of consensus and integrated efforts among professionals from different disciplines who are working on CFS.

In light of current knowledge limitations, treatment plans for CFS are interdisciplinary and holistic, and most patients include alternative therapies in their treatment plans. Empathy and compassion are essential components of providing care for CFS patients. CFS patients need the support and reassurance of their physicians to help them cope with their symptoms and resume normal, productive lives. The first and most important task for the health care professional is to develop mutual trust and collaboration with the patient. The second is to complete an adequate assessment, the aim of which is either to make a diagnosis of CFS or to identify an alternative cause for the patient's symptoms. The history is most important and should include a detailed account of the symptoms, the associated disability, the choice of coping strategies, and most important, the patient's own understanding of his or her illness. The assessment of possible comorbid psychiatric disorders, such as depression or anxiety, is mandatory. When the physician is satisfied that no alternative physical or psychiatric disorder can be found to explain symptoms, a diagnosis of CFS can be made. The treatment of CFS requires that the patient be given a positive explanation of the cause of his or her symptoms, emphasizing the distinction among factors that may have predisposed them to develop the illness (lifestyle, work stress, personality), triggered the illness (viral infection, life events), and perpetuated the illness (cerebral dysfunction, sleep disorder, depression, inconsistent activity, and misunderstanding of the illness and fear of making it worse). Interventions are then aimed to overcoming these illness-perpetuating factors.

Ciguatera: Chronic ciguatera can be confused with CFS.[1,2] Ciguatera is a distressing form of fish poisoning caused by the ingestion of one or more of a series of ciguatoxins. These poisons, some of the most potent mammalian neurotoxins known, are manufactured in reef-dwelling dinoflagellates and concentrated up the piscine food chain. Humans become poisoned by eating certain bottom-dwelling fish species. The acute intoxication is clinically dramatic, resulting in paresthesias, dysesthesias, prostration, myalgia, and arthralgia. In approximately 20 percent of cases, symptoms of fatigue, reduced exercise tolerance, and nonspecific headaches and pains persist for months and, in a small percentage of cases, for years. Occasionally, patients are encountered who have been diagnosed with CFS because of lack of awareness of the ciguatera syndrome, but in whom in retrospect the episode of acute fish poisoning can be established.[1,2]

Circadian rhythms: In one study,[1] CFS patients had circadian rhythms that were synchronous but of increased amplitudes, and systolic blood pressures consistently below 100 mm Hg during the nighttime (one hypertensive CFS patient was excluded). Although positive inotropic compounds may be beneficial in such patients as shown by a reduction in nighttime hypotension by inopamil (200 mg daily), melatonin (4 mg daily) increased nighttime hypotension. In a second study,[2] although there were no differences between the two groups in the amplitude, mean value or timing of the peak (acrophase) of the circardian rhythm of body core temperature or in the timing of the onset of melatonin secretion, CFS patients did not show the significant correlation between the timing of the temperature acrophase and the melatonin onset seen in controls. The latter dissociation of circadian rhythms can explain the finding of a study that used continuous 24-hour recordings of core body temperature, with an ingestible radio frequency transmitter pill and a belt-worn receiver-logger, and showed that CFS patients have normal core body temperatures despite frequent self-reports of subnormal body temperature and low-grade fever.[3] Dissociation of circadian rhythms could be secondary to the sleep deprivation and social disruption, and/or the reduction in physical activity that typically accompany CFS. By analogy with jet lag and shift working, circadian dysrhythmia could be an important factor in initiating and perpetuating the cardinal symptoms of CFS, notably tiredness, and impaired concentration and intellectual abilities.

Circulating immune complexes: Elevated levels of immune complexes have been reported in four studies,[1-4] while two other studies revealed no abnormality.[5,6] Depressed levels of complement[1,2,4-6] and elevated levels of C-reactive protein[7] have also been reported in up to 25 percent of CFS patients.

Cognitive behavioral therapy: Based on the notion that certain cognitions and behavior may perpetuate symptoms and disability, several studies addressed and supported the use of cognitive behavioral therapy in CFS.[1-13] In one study,[11] CFS patients underwent a comprehensive multidisciplinary intervention that included optimal medical management, pharmacologic treatment of any ongoing affective or anxiety disorder, and a comprehensive cognitive-behavioral treatment program. Of the 51 patients treated, 31 returned to gainful employment, 14 were functioning at a level equivalent to employment, and six remained significantly disabled. Follow-up at an average of 33 months later of a subgroup of treated patients showed good maintenance of gains. Untreated patients showed improvement in only a minority of cases. In a randomized control trial,[12] cognitive behavior therapy was more effective than a relaxation control in the management of CFS patients. Improvements were sustained over six months of follow-up. Another randomized control trial[13] showed that adding cognitive behavior therapy to the medical care of patients with CFS is acceptable to patients and leads to a sustained reduction in functional impairment. Illness beliefs and coping behavior previously associated with a poor outcome changed more with cognitive behavior therapy than with medical care alone. *See also* ILLNESS BELIEFS, NEUROPSYCHOLOGY, PERSONALITY TRAITS, PSYCHOPATHOLOGY.

Cognitive function: *See* NEUROPSYCHOLOGY.

Concentration: *See* NEUROPSYCHOLOGY.

Connective tissue and rheumatologic disorders: CFS has features of autoimmune diseases, a feature which may complicate diagnosis. For instance, three cases of dermatomyositis had been erroneously diagnosed as CFS because of the presence of elevated titers of serum Epstein-Barr virus antibodies.[1] In one study, one-third of CFS patients with sicca symptoms fulfilled the diagnostic criteria for Sjögren's syndrome, but they were "seronegative," differing from the ordinary primary Sjögren's syndrome.[2] An additional confounding feature is that patients with primary Sjögren's syndrome report more fatigue than healthy controls on all the dimensions of the Multidimensional Fatigue Inventory and, when controlling for depression, significant differences remain on the dimensions of general fatigue, physical fatigue, and reduced activity.[3] The negative correlation between levels of noradrenaline and general fatigue in patients with primary Sjögren's syndrome may imply the involvement of the autonomic nervous system in the chronic fatigue reported in this syndrome.[3,4] Although fatigue in patients with systemic lupus erythematosus (SLE) does not correlate with disease activity, it is correlated with fibromyalgia, depression, and lower overall health status.[5] Fatigue is also a major symptom in patients with ankylosing spondylitis and, unlike SLE, it is more likely to occur with active disease but it may occur as a lone symptom.[6] Fatigue is also common in osteoarthritis and rheumatoid arthritis, associates with measures of distress, and is a predictor of work dysfunction and overall health status.[7] Several studies[8,9] have reported that rheumatoid arthritis-related fatigue is strongly associated with psychosocial variables, apart from disease activity *per se*. Fatigue is associated to a large extent with pain, self-efficacy toward coping with disease, toward asking for help and problematic social support, and female gender. One study[10] found large individual differences in variation of pain and fatigue among rheumatoid arthritis patients. Stressors were associated with increased pain, but not fatigue. Subjects experiencing poor sleep had higher levels of pain and fatigue. Diurnal cycles of pain and fatigue were found, yet were observed for only some patients.

Coping: *See* ILLNESS BELIEFS, PERSONALITY TRAITS, PSYCHOPATHOLOGY.

Core body temperature: *See* CIRCADIAN RHYTHMS.

Coronary artery disease: No significant difference between CFS patients and controls can be found among risk factors for coronary artery disease (aerobic physical fitness, basic anthropometric data, blood pressure, spectrum of blood lipoproteins, blood uric acid, and smoking habits).[1] In non-CFS patients, it appears that the association of excess fatigue with atherosclerotic disease is largely associated with established risk factors, the most prominent of which is smoking.[2]

Corticotropin-releasing hormone (CRH): *See* NEUROENDOCRINOL-OGY.

Cortisol: *See* NEUROENDOCRINOLOGY.

Creatine: *See* NUTRITION.

Cyanocobalamin: *See* NUTRITION.

Cysteine: *See* LOW CYSTEINE-GLUTATHIONE SYNDROME.

Cytokines: Stimulated lymphoid cells either express or induce the expression in other cells of a heterogeneous group of soluble mediators that exhibit either effector or regulatory functions. These soluble mediators include cytokines, hormones, and neurotransmitters, which in turn affect immune function and may underlie many of the pathological manifestations seen in CFS.[1] The studies of cytokines in CFS have been done in the peripheral blood compartment and a recent review on the immunopathogenesis of CFS concludes that neuropsychiatric symptoms in CFS patients may be more closely related to disordered cytokine production by glial cells within the central nervous system (CNS) than to circulating cytokines.[2] The hypothesis that expression of proinflammatory cytokines within the CNS plays a role in the pathogenesis of immunologically-mediated fatigue is underscored by a study that used two strains of mice with differential patterns of cytokine expression in response to an injection challenge with *Corynebacterium parvum* and demonstrated elevated IL-1 and tumor necrosis factor (TNF) cytokine messenger ribonucleic acid (mRNA) expression in the

CNS in association with development of fatigue.[3] Systemic injection of antibodies specific to either IL-1 or TNF did not alter immunologically-induced fatigue, suggesting a lack of involvement of these cytokines produced outside of the CNS.[3]

The decreased natural killer cell cytotoxic and lymphoproliferative activities and increased allergic and autoimmune manifestations in CFS would be compatible with the hypothesis that the immune systems of affected individuals are biased toward a Th2 type, or humoral immunity-oriented cytokine pattern.[4] Although vaccines and stressful stimuli have been shown to lead to long-term, nonspecific shifts in cytokine balance, the factors that could lead to a Th2 shift in CFS patients are unknown. Nevertheless, therapeutic regimens, including repeated stimulation with bacterial antigens[5,6] and ex vivo activation of lymph node cells which induce a systemic Th1 bias, are being tested with preliminary success. *See also* INTERFERONS (IFNS), INTERLEUKIN-1 (IL-1) AND SOLUBLE IL-1 RECEPTORS, INTERLEUKIN-2 (IL-2) AND SOLUBLE IL-2 RECEPTOR, INTERLEUKIN-4 (IL-4), INTERLEUKIN-6 (IL-6) AND SOLUBLE IL-6 RECEPTOR, INTERLEUKIN-10 (IL-10), TUMOR GROWTH FACTOR BETA (TGF-beta), TUMOR NECROSIS FACTORS (TNFs) AND SOLUBLE TNF RECEPTORS.

Cytomegalovirus (CMV): *See* HERPESVIRUSES.

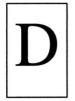

Daytime sleepiness: *See* SLEEP.

Demographics: Several studies have documented a female gender predominance in CFS. For instance, a study[1] of 118 questionnaires completed by members of the Irish College of General Practitioners yielded a male-to-female ratio of 1:2 with all social classes represented while a male-to-female ratio of 1:5 was found in a study[2] of 601 patients in four family practices in Leyden. The findings of one group[3,4] disagree with the female predominance reported in other studies: Diaries kept by Dutch citizens over a 21-day period showed that the majority of those with persistent fatigue complaints were male, middle-aged, less educated, and unemployed, and they had more psychological and psychosocial problems than the incidental fatigue sufferers. Moreover, a study[5] of primary care patients in

England found that rates of chronic fatigue and CFS did not vary by social class and that, after adjustment for psychological disorder, being female was modestly associated with chronic fatigue. The latter findings could be reconciled by a study[6] on the natural history of an outbreak in 1984 of an illness characterized by prolonged unexplained fatigue in West Otago, New Zealand, an outbreak that resembled other reported outbreaks of epidemic neuromyasthenia in that affected individuals presented with a spectrum of complaints ranging from transient diarrhea and upper respiratory disorders to CFS. The latter study revealed a female predominance among patients meeting the CDC case definition for CFS, whereas males predominated in patients diagnosed as having prolonged or idiopathic fatigue. Moreover, a comparison[7] of subjects fulfilling criteria for CFS, identified as part of a prospective cohort study in primary care, compared to adults fulfilling the same criteria referred for treatment to a specialist CFS clinic showed that although women were over-represented in both primary care and hospital groups, the high rates of psychiatric morbidity and female excess that characterize CFS in specialist settings are not due to selection bias. On the other hand, higher social class and physical illness attributions may be the result of selection bias and not intrinsic to CFS. A survey of 3,500 Norwegians, aged 18-90, revealed that although women were found to be more fatigued than men, no firm associations between fatigue and age or social variables could be found.[8] In contrast to the Norwegian experience, a cross-sectional telephone screening survey, followed by interviews of 8,004 households (16,970 residents) in San Francisco, revealed that chronic fatigue illnesses (CFS or idiopathic) were most prevalent among women, African Americans, Native Americans, persons engaged in clerical occupations, and persons with annual household incomes below $40,000, and least prevalent among Asians.[9]

Dental amalgam fillings: In a study of 99 self-referred patients complaining of multiple somatic and mental symptoms attributed to dental amalgam fillings, one-third of the patients reported symptoms of CFS compared with none of 80 in a dental control sample (patients with dental amalgam fillings seen in an ordinary dental practice) and only 2 and 6 percent, respectively, in the two clinical comparison samples (93 and 99 patients with known chronic medical disorders seen in alternative and ordinary medical family practices, respectively). The authors attributed the higher frequency of CFS symptomatology to the observation of higher mean neuroticism and lower lie scores in the dental amalgam group as compared to the comparison groups.[1] In contrast to the latter conclusion, another report described a patient who suffered from several complaints, which were attributed to her amalgam fillings, and analysis of mercury in plasma and urine showed unexpectedly high concentrations, 63 and 223 nmol/l, respectively. Following removal of the amalgam fillings, the urinary excretion of mercury became gradually normalized, and her symptoms declined.[2]

Depression: *See* PSYCHOPATHOLOGY.

Dermatomyositis: *See* CONNECTIVE TISSUE AND RHEUMATOLOGIC DISORDERS.

Dexamethasone: *See* NEUROENDOCRINOLOGY.

Dieting disorders: *See* PSYCHOPATHOLOGY.

Disability: CFS is associated with considerable personal and occupational disability and low rates of employment.[1,2] The potentially large economic burden of this disorder underscores the need for accurate estimates of direct and indirect costs, the relative contribution of individual factors to disability, and the need to develop targeted rehabilitation programs. The Medical Outcomes Study Short-Form General Health Survey (SF-36) is useful in assessing functional status in patients with fatiguing illnesses. In one study,[3] patients with CFS and chronic fatigue were found to have marked impairment of their functional status. The severity and pattern of impairment as documented by the SF-36 distinguishes patients with CFS and chronic fatigue (lowest scores) from those with major depression and acute infectious mononucleosis (intermediate scores), and from controls (highest scores), but does not discriminate between chronic fatigue and CFS patients. A large study[4] showed that CFS patients had marked impairment in comparison with the general population and disease comparison groups with hypertension, congestive heart failure, type II diabetes mellitus, acute myocardial infarction, multiple sclerosis, and depression. Moreover, the degree and pattern of impairment was different from that seen in patients with depression: CFS patients scored significantly lower on all SF-36 scales except for scales measuring mental health and role disability due to emotional problems, on which they scored significantly higher. The relationship in CFS between cognitive impairment and functional disability cannot be explained entirely on the basis of psychiatric factors.[5]

Energy expenditure: A study[1] measured resting energy expenditure by indirect calorimetry and measurement of total body potassium in 11 women with CFS and in 11 healthy women, and found that five out of the 11 CFS subjects had resting energy expenditure above the upper limit of normal as defined by the control group data. These findings were suggested to be consistent with an up-regulation of the sodium-potassium pump in CFS. Possible abnormalities in ion channel metabolism in CFS are being investigated by the same group of researchers.

Enteroviruses: Enteroviruses (Coxsackie A and B, echovirus, poliovirus) belong to a group of small RNA-viruses, picornavirus, that are widespread in nature. Enteroviruses cause a number of well-known diseases and symptoms in humans, from subclinical infections and the common cold to poliomyelitis with paralysis. Serologic and molecular biology techniques have demonstrated that enteroviral genomes, in certain situations, persist after the primary infection (which is often silent). Persistent enteroviral infection or recurrent infections and/or virus-stimulated autoimmunity might contribute to the development of diseases with hitherto unexplained pathogenesis, such as post-polio syndrome, dilated cardiomyopathy, juvenile (type 1) diabetes, and possibly some cases diagnosed as CFS.[1-3] Several studies have failed to document persistent enteroviral infections in CFS.[4-6] *See also* POST-POLIO SYNDROME.

Environmental chemicals: *See* MULTIPLE CHEMICAL SENSITIVITY (MCS) SYNDROME.

Eosinophils: *See* ALLERGIES.

Epidemiology: Epidemiologic studies of CFS have been hampered by the absence of a specific diagnostic test, but with increasing interest in this disorder there has been a greater understanding of the risk factors, illness patterns, and other aspects of this multisystem disorder. Working case definitions have been developed for research purposes, but they have continued to change over time and have not always been utilized precisely by various investigators. This has been a major factor in the widely varying estimates of prevalence rates,[1] but two different studies using the same working definition and including a medical work-up have estimated the prevalence to be approximately 200/100,000.[2] A study of the epidemiology of chronic debilitating fatigue based on questionnaires completed by members of the Irish College of General Practitioners yielded an estimated 2.1 cases per practice and an incidence of one per 1,000 population.[3] In a study of 214 primary care patients in England,[4] the point prevalence of chronic fatigue was 11.3 percent, falling to 4.1 percent if comorbid psychological disorders were excluded. The point prevalence of CFS was 2.6 percent, falling to 0.5 percent if comorbid psychological disorders were excluded. The prevalence of CFS based on a study of 601 patients in four family practices in Leyden was estimated to be at least 1.1 per 1,000 patients.[5] Extrapolation of the results from a study[6] based on questionnaires filled out by general practitioners indicates that there are at least 17,000 CFS patients in the Netherlands. The prevalence of CFS in teenagers is 10 to 20 per 100,000 inhabitants in the Netherlands.[7] A nationwide survey[8] conducted using the Japanese version of the CDC criteria for CFS in all clinical departments of internal medicine, pediatrics, psychiatry, and neurology at university hospitals and at ordinary hospitals with 200 or more beds yielded a period prevalence adjusted for a response rate of 0.85 (0.63 for males and 1.02 for females) per 100,000 population and a response adjusted incidence estimate of 0.46 per 100,000 person-years.

Clusters of CFS cases, which appear to be related to earlier reports of "epidemic neuromyasthenia," have attracted considerable attention and appear to be well documented, although investigated with varying methodology and often with dissimilar case definitions.[2,8] Risk factors for cases occurring in clusters and sporadically appear to be similar, the most consistent ones being female gender and the coexistence of some form of stress, either physical or psychological.[2] In a study[9] of an outbreak in 1984 of an illness characterized by prolonged unexplained fatigue was reported in West Otago, New Zealand, 23 of the 28 patients in the original report were contacted and ten (48 percent) of the 21 patients with satisfactory interviews appeared to meet the current CDC case definition of CFS, and 11 were classified as having prolonged or idiopathic fatigue. Not all cluster cases have been confirmed. For instance, data[10] collected from 1,698 households in four rural Michigan communities did not confirm a reported cluster of cases resembling CFS. The prevalence of households containing at least one fatigued person was similar between communities thought to harbor the cluster and communities selected for comparison.

In terms of possible infectious or environmental etiologies of CFS, a prospective cohort study[11] of 250 primary care patients revealed a higher incidence and longer duration of an acute fatigue syndrome, and a higher prevalence of CFS, after glandular fever versus an ordinary upper respiratory tract infection. A conservative estimate is that glandular fever accounts for 3,113 (95 percent CI 1,698-4,528) new cases of CFS per annum in England and Wales. In another study[12] based on data collected on two samples of nurses recruited through mailed questionnaires, a physician review team estimated the prevalence of CFS to be 1,088 per 100,000 among these health care professionals. These findings suggest that nurses might represent a high-risk group for this illness, possibly due to occupational stressors (exposure to viruses, shift schedules, and other stressors). Other studies disagree with the latter conclusion. *See* OCCUPATIONAL MEDICINE.

Epstein-Barr virus (EBV): *See* HERPESVIRUSES.

Exercise: CFS patients show a specific sensitivity to the effects of exertion on effortful cognitive functioning (focused and sustained attention).[1] After physically demanding exercise, CFS subjects demonstrate impaired cognitive processing (as assessed by the Symbol Digit Modalities Test, Stroop Word Test, and Stroop Color Test) compared with healthy individuals.[2] The observation that the performance decrements, associated with the development of CFS in an elite ultra-endurance athlete, were the result of detraining rather than an impairment of aerobic metabolism may be indicative of central, possibly neurological, factors influencing fatigue perception in CFS sufferers.[3] In this respect, a study[4] of the effects of exercise on motor evoked potentials elicited by transcranial magnetic stimulation found that postexercise cortical excitability is significantly reduced in patients with CFS and in depressed patients compared with that of normal subjects.

Although many CFS patients experience "relapses" of severe symptoms following even moderate levels of exertion, most studies report CFS patients to have normal muscle strength and either normal or slightly reduced muscle endurance.[5] Histological and metabolic studies report mixed results: CFS patients have either no impairment or mild impairment of mitochondria and oxidative metabolism compared with sedentary controls.[5] Measurement of physical activity after strenuous exercise in women with CFS compared to sedentary healthy volunteers who exercised no more than once per week revealed that although marked exertion produces changes in activity, these changes are apparent later than self-reports would suggest and they are not so severe that CFS patients cannot compensate.[6] One study[7] found that, compared with normal controls, women with CFS have an aerobic power indicating a low normal fitness level with no indication of cardiopulmonary abnormality. The CFS group could withstand a maximal treadmill exercise test without a major exacerbation in either fatigue or other symptoms of their illness. In cancer patients, for instance, exercise is a feasible and potentially beneficial intervention to combat distressing cancer treatment-related fatigue.[8] Several groups consider that exercise training programs are beneficial (if "relapses" can be avoided) in CFS, although few controlled studies have been performed.[9-18] A randomized controlled trial[9] to test the efficacy of a graded aerobic exercise program in 66 CFS patients with control treatment crossover after the first follow-up examination supports the use of appropriately prescribed graded aerobic exercise in the management of CFS patients.

Familial chronic fatigue syndrome: A study of natural killer (NK) cell activity in a family with members who had developed CFS as adults, as compared to those who had not, documented low NK activity in six out of eight cases and in four out of twelve unaffected family members. Two of the offspring of the CFS cases had pediatric malignancies. Based on these observations, the authors suggest that the low NK cell activity in this family may be a result of a genetically determined immunologic abnormality predisposing to CFS and cancer.[1,2]

Fatigue: Although fatigue is probably the most common symptom of illness affecting sufferers of both acute and chronic conditions, it is also a universal complaint that may or may not be related to medical diagnoses or therapeutic treatments.[1-6] Therefore, confusion surrounds the definition and use of the term fatigue. As with many other medical concepts, it is a word that is commonly used in colloquial language. Fatigue is a complex, multicausal, multidimensional, nonspecific, and subjective phenomenon for which no one definition is widely accepted. The condition of fatigue requires adequate assessments, innovative planning and interventions, and patient-centered evaluations by healthcare professionals. Fatigue, whether acute or chronic, needs to be recognized as a true and valid condition in order for treatment to be successful. Chronic fatigue and acute fatigue can be quite different conditions, requiring different approaches.[1-6] *See also* ACQUIRED IMMUNODEFICIENCY SYNDROME (AIDS) AND FATIGUE, BRAIN INJURY AND FATIGUE, CANCER AND FATIGUE, CHRONIC FATIGUE SYNDROME (CFS), DEFINITION, CONNECTIVE TISSUE AND RHEUMATOLOGIC DISORDERS, POST-DIALYSIS FATIGUE.

Fibromyalgia: Fibromyalgia is a form of nonarticular rheumatism characterized by musculoskeletal aching, tenderness on palpation, and systemic symptoms.[1-5] Nearly all rheumatologists now accept fibromyalgia as a distinct diagnostic entity. In fact, in the United States it is the third or fourth most common reason for rheumatology referral.[3] Fibromyalgia symptoms last, on average, at least 15 years after illness onset. However, most patients experience some improvement in symptoms before that time.[6] Patients with fibromyalgia report greater difficulty in performing activities of daily living as well as increased pain, fatigue, and weakness compared with healthy controls.[1-6] Measurements of P-31 magnetic resonance spectroscopy (MRS)[7] show that patients have significantly lower than normal phosphocreatine and adenosine triphosphate (ATP) levels and phosphocreatine/inorganic phosphate ratios in the quadriceps muscles during rest. Values for phosphorylation potential and total oxidative capacity also were significantly reduced during rest and exercise.

There is clinical and, in many cases, demographic overlap between fibromyalgia, CFS, and syndromes including neurally mediated hypotension, abnormalities of the growth hormone-insulin-like growth factor-1 axis, and the presence of autoantibodies.[8-14] Although the role of psychological factors in fibromyalgia has been controversial,[15-19] anxiety and depression are independently associated with severity of pain symptoms in fibromyalgia[20] and, in one report, the presence of multiple lifetime psychiatric diagnoses was not intrinsically related to fibromyalgia, but rather to the decision of patients to seek specialty medical care.[9] Disability among children with fibromyalgia is also a function of a child's psychological adjustment and physical state, and of a parent's physical state and method of coping with pain.[19]

Treatment of patients with fibromyalgia and CFS continues to be of limited success, although the role of multidisciplinary group intervention appears promising.[1-5] A study showed that although short-term treatment (16 nights) with zolpidem (5 to 15 mg at bedtime) does not affect the pain of fibromyalgia, it is useful for sleep and daytime energy in this patient population.[21] Administration of gamma-hydroxybutyrate in divided doses at night in 11 fibromyalgia patients resulted in significant improvement in both fatigue and pain, with an increase in slow wave sleep and a decrease in the severity of the alpha anomaly.[22]

Folic acid: *See* NUTRITION.

Fluoxetine: *See* SELECTIVE SEROTONIN REUPTAKE INHIBITORS (SSRIs).

Food intolerance: *See* ALLERGIES.

Gait: *See* NEUROPHYSIOLOGY.

Gastric emptying: *See* GASTROINTESTINAL PATHOLOGY.

Gastrointestinal pathology: Patients with CFS or fibromyalgia with or without chronic facial pain show a high comorbidity with irritable bowel syndrome, an observation that may reflect a shared underlying pathophysiologic basis involving dysregulation of the hypothalamic-pituitary-adrenal stress hormone axis in predisposed individuals.[1-5] Although the etiologies of irritable bowel syndrome and chronic fatigue are unknown, psychological as well as physical factors have been implicated in both, and fatigue is common in irritable bowel syndrome patients. Although a subgroup of patients with irritable bowel syndrome may also have CFS, the two diagnoses should be considered separately.[1-5] In this respect, normal gastric emptying and myoelectrical activity were found in adolescents with CFS.[6]

Gender: *See* DEMOGRAPHICS.

Glandular fever: A prospective cohort study[1] of 250 primary care patients in England revealed a higher incidence and longer duration of an acute fatigue syndrome, and a higher prevalence of CFS, after glandular fever versus an ordinary upper respiratory tract infection. The authors estimated that glandular fever accounts for 3,113 (95 percent CI 1,698-4,528) new cases of CFS per annum in England and Wales. New episodes of major depressive disorder were triggered by infection, especially the Epstein-Barr virus, but lasted a median of only three weeks. No psychiatric disorder was significantly more prevalent six months after onset than before. A second study[2] by the same group found that the ability to process information after glandular fever or an ordinary upper respiratory tract infection is related to estimates of premorbid IQ, whereas poor concentration is related independently to both psychiatric morbidity and a fatigue state, but not the particular infection itself. *See also* NEUROPSYCHOLOGY.

Glucocorticoids: *See* NEUROENDOCRINOLOGY.

Glutamine/L-Glutamine: *See* NUTRITION.

Glutathione: *See* LOW CYSTEINE-GLUTATHIONE SYNDROME.

Glycogen: *See* NUTRITION.

Glyconutrients: *See* NUTRITION.

Growth hormone (GH): *See* ACQUIRED IMMUNODEFICIENCY SYNDROME (AIDS) AND FATIGUE, NEUROENDOCRINOLOGY.

Gulf War syndrome: A study[1] of 3,695 military personnel found that those who participated in the Persian Gulf War had a higher self-reported prevalence of medical and psychiatric conditions than contemporary military personnel who were not deployed to the Persian Gulf. Compared with non-Persian Gulf War military personnel, Persian Gulf War military personnel reported a significantly higher prevalence of symptoms of depression, post-traumatic stress disorder (PTSD), chronic fatigue, cognitive dysfunction, bronchitis, asthma, fibromyalgia, alcohol abuse, anxiety, and sexual discomfort. Assessment of health-related quality of life demonstrated diminished mental and physical functioning scores for Persian Gulf War military personnel. The New Jersey Center for Environmental Hazards Research[2] found that more than half of the Persian Gulf Registry veterans reported illness characterized by severe fatigue and symptoms consistent with chemical sensitivities. Human challenge testing procedures will allow testing of theories of causal relationships of airborne allergens and chemicals with allergic sensitization potential and the causal relationship of chemical exposure and the Persian Gulf War syndrome.[3-6] One report[7] suggests that the symptoms of Persian Gulf War syndrome are compatible with the hypothesis that the immune system of affected individuals is biased toward a Th2 (humoral immunity-oriented)-cytokine pattern. Factors that could lead to a Th2 shift among Gulf War veterans include exposure to multiple vaccinations, most of which are Th2-inducing under stressful circumstances and the way in which such vaccinations were administered, which would be expected to maximize Th2 immunogenicity. These factors may have led to a long-term systemic shift toward a Th2-cytokine balance and to mood changes related to the immunoendocrine state. Other vaccines that lead to similar long-term, nonspecific shifts in cytokine balance are well established.[7] Some authors contend that because Armed Forces Reserve members, especially combat support units, were rapidly mobilized during Operation Desert Shield/Desert Storm, they were at higher risk for anxiety and stress-related disorders which may have contributed to the development of later symptoms.[8]

Gynecology: A case-control study[1] analyzed data collected in self-administered questionnaires on menstrual, reproductive, and medical histories of 149 women being seen for nongynecologic conditions with and without CFS. Women with CFS reported increased gynecologic complications and a lower incidence of premenstrual symptomatology, both of which could be explained by the higher number of self-reported cases of irregular cycles, periods of amenorrhea, and sporadic bleeding between menstrual periods, and the higher frequency of histories of polycystic ovarian syndrome, hirsutism, and ovarian cysts among women with CFS as compared to controls.

Heart rate variability: *See* AUTONOMIC FUNCTION.

Herpesviruses: Herpesviruses (Epstein-Barr virus, cytomegalovirus, human herpesvirus types 6 and 7, herpes simplex virus types 1 and 2) have been associated with CFS. For instance, reactivation/replication of a latent herpesvirus (such as Epstein-Barr virus) could modulate the immune system to induce CFS.[1] In this respect, serologically proven acute infectious illness due to Epstein-Barr virus (EBV) is associated with a range of nonspecific somatic and psychological symptoms, particularly fatigue and malaise rather than anxiety and depression.[2] Although improvement in several symptoms occurs rapidly, fatigue commonly remains a prominent complaint at four weeks, and resolution of fatigue is associated with improvement in cell-mediated immunity. A prospective cohort study[3] of 250 primary care patients also revealed a higher incidence and longer duration of an acute fatigue syndrome, and a higher prevalence of CFS, after glandular fever as compared to after an ordinary upper respiratory tract infection. In another study,[4] anti-EBV titers were higher among CFS patients and were associated with being more symptomatic. However, testing[5] of 548 chronically fatigued patients, including patients with CFS, for antibodies to 13 viruses (herpes simplex virus 1 and 2, rubella, adenovirus, human herpesvirus 6, Epstein-Barr virus, cytomegalovirus (CMV), and Coxsackie B virus, types 1-6 in patients) found no consistent differences in any of the seroprevalences compared with controls.

Cloned DNA obtained from the culture of an African green monkey simian cytomegalovirus-derived stealth virus contains multiple discrete regions of significant sequence homology to portions of known human cellular genes.[6] The stealth virus has also been cultured from several CFS patients and a cytopathic stealth virus was also cultured from the cerebrospinal fluid of a nurse with CFS. The findings lend support to the possibility of replicative RNA forms of certain stealth viruses.[7] Review[8] of the clinical histories and brain biopsy findings of three patients with severe stealth virus encephalopathy showed that the patients initially developed symptoms consistent with CFS. One patient has remained in a vegetative state for several years, while the other two patients have shown significant, although incomplete, recovery. Histological and electron-microscopic studies revealed vacuolated cells with distorted nuclei and various cytoplasmic inclusions suggestive of incomplete viral expression. No significant inflammatory response occurred. Viral cultures provided further evidence of stealth viral infections occurring in these patients.[8] Partial sequencing[9] of stealth virus segments isolated from a CFS patient revealed a fragmented genome and sequence microheterogeneity, which suggested that both the processivity and the fidelity of replication of the viral genome were defective. An unstable viral genome may provide a potential mechanism of recovery from stealth viral illness.

Some studies suggest an association between human herpesvirus-6 (HHV-6) (roseolovirus genus of the betaherpesvirus subfamily) and CFS.[10-13] One study found that a high proportion (50 percent by antibody testing and up to 80 percent by nested-polymerase chain reaction (PCR) detection of viral DNA but not RNA) of CFS patients were infected with HHV-6, but with low viral load. The latter results do not support HHV-6 reactivation in CFS patients.[13]

Use of the supernatant fluid from HHV-7 infected cells as antigen in immunoassays yielded high and low HHV-7 antibody in sera from chronic fatigue patients and healthy donors as controls, respectively.[14]

Transfer factors (TF) with specific activity against herpesviruses have been documented in CFS. With some studies suggesting that persistent viral activity may play a role in perpetuation of CFS symptoms, there appears to be a rationale for the use of TF in patients with CFS, and recent reports have suggested that transfer factors may play a beneficial role in this disorder.[15-18] For instance, specific HHV-6 TF preparation, administered to two CFS patients, inhibited the HHV-6 infection.[16] Prior to treatment, both patients exhibited an activated HHV-6 infection. TF treatment significantly improved the clinical manifestations of CFS in one patient who resumed normal duties within weeks, whereas no clinical improvement was observed in the second patient. Of the 20 patients in a placebo-controlled trial of oral TF,[17] improvement was observed in 12 patients, generally within three to six weeks of beginning treatment. However, in this study herpesvirus serology (EBV and HHV-6) seldom correlated with clinical response. Treatment with TF of a group of 222 patients suffering from cellular immunodeficiency (CID), frequently combined with CFS and/or chronic viral infections by EBV and/or cytomegalovirus (CMV),[18] showed that age, but not gender, substantially influenced the failure rate of CID treatment using TF. In older people, it is easier to improve the clinical condition than CID. This may be related to the diminished number of lymphocytes; however, a placebo effect cannot be totally excluded.

HLA-DR: *See* LYMPHOCYTES.

Hirsutism: *See* GYNECOLOGY.

Homocysteine: One study found that increased homocysteine levels in the central nervous system characterize patients fulfilling the criteria for both CFS and fibromyalgia. A significant positive correlation occurred between both high cerebrospinal fluid (CSF)-homocysteine and low CSF-B12 levels and fatigability. Vitamin B12 deficiency causes a deficient remethylation of homocysteine and therefore probably contributed to the increased homocysteine levels found.[1] *See also* NUTRITION.

Human herpesvirus-6 (HHV-6): *See* HERPESVIRUSES.

Human herpesvirus-7 (HHV-7): *See* HERPESVIRUSES.

Hydrocortisone: *See* NEUROENDOCRINOLOGY.

Hyperventilation: *See* REGULATION OF RESPIRATION.

Hypothalamus-pituitary-adrenal (HPA) axis: *See* NEUROENDO-CRINOLOGY.

Hypothyroidism: Although hypothyroidism with a modest elevation of thyroid-stimulating hormone has been reported in approximately 7 percent of CFS cases[1-6] and several studies have documented the presence of antithyroid antibodies,[7-9] CFS patients usually remained fatigued after correction of their hypothyroidism.[2] Interleukin-1 (IL-1) inhibits thyrotropin release,[10] and several cytokines, including IL-1,[10] IL-6, and IFN-α,[11] have been shown to be cytotoxic to thyroid cells, properties which could mediate the hypothyroidism seen in some CFS cases. In this respect, fatigue occurs in more than 70 percent of patients treated with interferon-alpha (IFN-alpha) and may be associated with the development of immune-mediated endocrine diseases, in particular hypothryoidism and hypothalamic-pituitary-adrenal axis-related hormonal deficiencies.[11] *See also* THYROXINE.

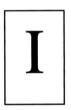

Iceland disease: Iceland disease or Akureyri disease is characterized by prolonged chronic fatigue that results in anxiety disorders following infection. The more serious psychiatric disorders (agoraphobia with panic attacks, agoraphobia without panic attacks, social phobia, simple phobia, schizophrenia, and alcohol dependence) do not seem to play a major role in the long run.[1]

Illness beliefs: The literature on the role of illness beliefs/attributions on the part of both patients and health care professionals is widely divided and some have gone as far as suggesting that chronic fatigue is merely a question of attribution.[1-3] The findings in a study[4] of 60 CFS patients suggested that physical illness attributions were less important in determining outcome (at least in treatment studies), and that good outcome was associated with change in avoidance behavior and related beliefs, rather than causal attributions. Another study[5] of 137 CFS patients concluded that the belief that one's actions can influence outcomes modified the relationship between illness accommodation and both fatigue and impairment; adverse outcomes were associated with accommodating to illness only in the context of lower levels of perceived control. It was suggested, therefore, that interventions that either discourage avoidance of activity or enhance perceived control could benefit the course of the illness. A series of regression analyses in one study[6] showed illness representations to be stronger predictors of adaptive outcome than coping scores.

Some studies emphasize the patient's attributions of disease as the cause for symptomatology. For instance, a study[7] of 153 women from the Toronto area who were attending a women's health symposium yielded an overwhelming endorsement of social determinants as the cause of their persistent fatigue. Although depression and anxiety formed the most robust associations with persistent fatigue in primary care and community studies, women in this sample ranked these factors in seventh place in their attributions. Similarly, although physicians often assume physical causes for fatigue, women rank physical health low in their own attributions. A study[8] comparing medical records of 133 CFS and 75 multiple sclerosis permanent health insurance claimants and 162 nonclaimant controls cases showed that CFS patients recorded significantly more illnesses at time of proposal for insurance than the two control groups, and had significantly more claims between proposal and diagnosis of their disorder. These observations led the authors to conclude that there is no support for a specific viral or immunological explanation for CFS and that abnormal illness behavior is of great importance.

Other studies have emphasized the role of the physician in disease perpetuation. For instance, a study[9] of 2,097 individuals in the Netherlands found that more psychosocially attributed fatigue was found to correlate with consultations characterized by less physical examination, more diagnostic procedures to reassure, fewer diagnostic procedures to discover underlying pathology, more counseling, less medical treatment, less prescription, and a longer duration than consultations with more somatically attributed fatigue. The study concluded that general practitioners do not discriminate between social groups when attributing fatigue to either somatic or psychosocial causes. The presence and character of other complaints and underlying diseases/problems, rather, relate to the general practitioners' somatic psychosocial attributions, which are then associated with particular aspects of the consultation. Research in one study[10] of 609 CFS patients suggested several patterns of relationships between doctors and patients, and attitudes to health and illness, which may alert doctors to patients' perceptions, beliefs, encoded constructs, and patterns of relating that affect responses to treatment. The study suggested that more attention from doctors to patients who are experiencing the stress of chronic illness is indicated. The latter view is reinforced by another study[11] that found that CFS patients complained about insufficient informational as well as emotional support from their doctors and, as a consequence, most opted for alternative or complementary forms of treatment. In addition, disagreements over illness etiology and treatment precluded effective cooperation.

Some studies have addressed the influence of illness attributions by family members on the disease process. A study[12] of adolescents with CFS in the Netherlands concluded that factors contributing to the persistence of fatigue are somatic attributions, illness-enhancing cognitions, and behavior of parents as well as physical inactivity. The role of the physician and the role of parents can enhance the problems. The treatment should focus on decreasing the somatic attributions, on reinforcement by the parents of healthy adolescent behavior, on the gradual increase of physical activity, and on decreasing attention (including medical attention) for the somatic complaints. A women's study[13] showed that some women respondents were able to identify specific ways in which family and important others could help them to decrease or prevent their fatigue. However, many expressed the belief that significant others were unconcerned and unwilling to assist them in any substantive way. Analysis of responses in one study[14] of 66 CFS participants indicated that, whereas the most commonly described explanation for the illness was a physical one, more than half the patients also believed "stress" had played a role. Patients believed that they could partially control the symptoms by reducing activity, but felt helpless to influence the physical disease process and hence the course of the illness. Patients reported that they had arrived at these beliefs about the illness after prolonged reflection on their own experiences combined with the reading of media reports, self-help books, and patient group literature. The views of health professionals played a relatively small role.

In conclusion, attribution contributes to the course of CFS, but it is not its sole determinant.[15] The presence of strong somatic attributions appears to be one of the perpetuating factors in CFS, but not the only one. Many CFS patients present a self-diagnosis. Communication problems between patient and doctor easily arise because of different attributions of the complaints. At the start of fatigue, somatic attributions are of less importance than later on in the course of the complaints. In this process, an iatrogenic factor might be involved. On the other hand, doctors are able to influence these attributions actively in a favorable direction.

Immune cell phenotypic distributions: Analysis of the complex interactions underlying immune responses was greatly facilitated by the development of monoclonal antibodies to various surface proteins on lymphoid cells, which defined functionally distinct subsets.[1-2] Such analysis has also demonstrated that each type of lymphoid cell is genetically programmed to carry out defined immunological functions that are predictable on the basis of surface phenotype.[3]

Surface-marker phenotyping of peripheral blood lymphoid cells has also allowed insight into the cellular basis of immune dysfunction associated with pathologies of the central nervous system with diverse causes, including viral, autoimmune, and genetic, among others.[3-10] Several reports also documented alterations in the distribution of various lymphoid cell subsets among CFS patients. Certain discrepancies in the findings from different study groups can be attributed to group nonequivalences on diverse parameters such as demographic variables (gender, age, socioeconomic status), medical status variables predating onset of disease, medication use, concomitant substance abuse, nutritional status, and the effects of time of sample collection (diurnal or seasonal variations).[5,11-18] *See* LYMPHOCYTES, NATURAL KILLER (NK) CELLS.

Immunoglobulins: Spontaneous and mitogen-induced immunoglobulin synthesis is depressed in 10 percent of patients with CFS.[1-3] The latter decrease may be a result of an increased T-cell suppression of immunoglobulin synthesis because a similar effect is obtained *in vitro* when using normal allogeneic B cells.[3] This inhibitory effect may also account for the reported difficulty in establishing spontaneous outgrowth of EBV-transformed B-cell lines from cells from CFS patients.[3-5] The depletion of the CD4+CD45RA+ lymphocyte subset in two studies may be associated with alteration in B-cell regulation.[6,7]

In 12 studies, CFS patients were found to have decreased amounts of immunoglobulins of the G, A, M, or D classes;[3-5,8-16] in five studies no difference was found;[17-21] and in one study IgG levels were elevated whereas IgA levels were normal.[22] IgG subclass deficiency, particularly of the opsonins IgG1 or IgG3, can be demonstrated in a substantial percentage of CFS patients,[6,11,13,16,23,24] and for a subset of these, immunoglobulin replacement therapy may be beneficial[25-28] albeit controversial.[29] One study failed to find immunoglobulin subclass deficiencies in CFS patients.[30] *See also* AUTOIMMUNITY.

Inflammatory bowel disease: *See* GASTROINTESTINAL PATHOLOGY.

Information processing: *See* NEUROPSYCHOLOGY.

Inner ear disorders: Twenty-eight of 80 patients with sudden deafness and progressive hearing losses (approximately half of whom had phospholipid antibodies that can cause venous or arterial vasculopathies, or serotonin and ganglioside antibodies) displayed symptoms typical for fibromyalgia and chronic fatigue disorders including fatigue, myalgia, arthralgia, depressions, sicca symptoms, and diarrhea.[1] The authors recommend questioning patients suffering from inner ear disorders for symptoms typical for fibromyalgia or CFS, since these diseases are often closely related to inner ear disorders. If symptoms are present, antibodies should be tested against phospholipids, serotonin, and gangliosides.

Inomapil: *See* CIRCADIAN RHYTHMS.

Insulin-like growth factors (IGFs): *See* NEUROENDOCRINOLOGY.

Interferons (IFNs): The IFNs comprise a multigenic family with pleiotropic properties and diverse cellular origin. Data from six studies indicated that circulating IFNs were present in 3 percent or less of patients studied.[1-7]

Peripheral blood cells from children affected by postviral fatigue syndrome produced more IFN-alpha than those from controls (Lever et al. 1988).[8] In line with the latter observation, one group found elevated IFN-alpha levels in CFS patients,[9] but two other groups found no difference.[10,11] Fatigue occurs in more than 70 percent of patients treated with IFN-alpha and it may be associated with the development of immune-mediated endocrine diseases, in particular hypothryoidism and hypothalamic-pituitary-adrenal axis-related hormonal deficiencies, in these patients.[12,13] IFN-alpha therapy-associated fatigue is often the dominant dose-limiting side effect, worsening with continued therapy, and accompanied by significant depression. Although the direct cause of IFN-alpha-induced fatigue is unknown, it is possible that neuromuscular fatigue, similar to that observed in patients with post-polio syndrome, may also be one component of this syndrome. The induction of proinflammatory cytokines observed in patients treated with IFN-alpha is consistent with a possible mechanism of neuromuscular pathology that could manifest as fatigue. A study also revealed that IFN-alpha/beta is at least partially responsible for the early fatigue induced by polyI:C during prolonged treadmill running in mice.[14]

IFN-gamma is an immunoregulatory substance, enhancing both cellular antigen presentation to lymphocytes[15] and natural killer cell cytotoxicity,[16] and causing inhibition of suppressor T lymphocyte activity.[17] Two groups have found impaired IFN-gamma production on mitogenic stimulation of peripheral blood mononuclear cells from CFS patients[18,19] and one group found increased production.[20] In contrast with the findings on lymphocyte activation, four groups reported no difference in the levels of circulating IFN-gamma.[10,11,19,21] These results are in favor of the Th2 shift described previously (*see* CYTO-KINES), a shift that is not always apparent at the level of circulating cytokines.

Interleukin-1 (IL-1) and soluble IL-1 receptors: IL-1 is the term for two distinct cytokines—IL-1α and IL-1β—that share the same cell-surface receptors and biological activities.[1,2] One study of CFS patients found elevated levels of serum IL-1 alpha, but not of plasma IL-1 beta in 17 percent of patients studied.[3] When the cohort was examined as to severity of symptoms, it was noted that the top quartile in terms of disability had the highest level of IL-1. Curiously, use of reverse transcriptase-coupled polymerase chain reaction (RT-PCR) revealed IL-1β, but not IL-1α messenger RNA (mRNA) in peripheral blood mononuclear cells (PBMCs) of several CFS patients with highly elevated levels of IL-1α. RT-PCR of fractionated cell populations showed that lymphocytes accounted for the IL-1β mRNA detected in PBMCs. No IL-1 mRNA was apparent in control subjects. That IL-1α mRNA was not detectable by RT-PCR in either PBMCs or granulocytes suggests that serum IL-1α in CFS patients is probably derived from a source other than peripheral blood cells. Other potential sources are tissue macrophages, endothelial cells, lymph node cells, fibroblasts, central nervous system microglia, astrocytes, and dermal dendritic cells.[1]

Although one group found significantly higher levels of IL-1 alpha in CFS and mononucleosis patients,[4] three other groups found no difference.[5-7] Five studies, in addition to the one described above,[6] found no difference in the levels of IL-1 beta in CFS patients.[4,6-9]

The signs and symptoms of CFS, which include fatigue, myalgia, and low-grade fever, are similar to those experienced by patients infused with cytokines such as interleukin-1. Elevated serum levels of IL-1α found in a significant number of CFS patients could underlie several of the clinical symptoms. IL-1 can gain access to the brain through the preoptic nucleus of the hypothalamus, where it induces fever and the release of adrenocorticotropin hormone (ACTH)-releasing factor,[10-13] which in turn would lead to release of ACTH and cortisol. The observation that cortisol levels tend to be low in CFS patients regardless of IL-1α levels suggests a role of a defective hypothalamic feedback loop in the pathogenesis of CFS. The presence of such a defect has been documented in Lewis rats, which are particularly susceptible to the induction of a variety of inflammatory and autoimmune diseases, and exhibit reduced levels of ACTH-releasing factor, ACTH, and cortisol in response to IL-1.

Besides its effects on the hypothalamus-pituitary-adrenal (HPA) axis, IL-1 has other effects on the pituitary; it has been shown to augment release of prolactin and growth hormone and to inhibit release of thyrotropin and luteinizing hormone.[14,15] The growth hormone deficiency state associated with CFS may also be a reflection of the defect in the hypothalamic feedback loop that renders it inadequately responsive to IL-1. *See* NEUROENDOCRINOLOGY.

IL-1 and tumor necrosis factor (TNF) provoke slow-wave sleep when placed in the lateral ventricles of experimental animals.[16] The inordinate fatigue, lassitude, and excessive sleepiness associated with CFS[17,18] could well be a consequence of the direct action of these cytokines on neurons.

IL-1 induces prostaglandin (PGE_2, PGI_2) synthesis by endothelial and smooth muscle cells.[19] These substances are potent vasoldilators, and IL-1 administration in animals and humans produces significant hypotension. IL-1 has a natriuretic effect[20] and may affect plasma volume.

IL-1 and TNF inhibit β-adrenergic agonist-mediated cardiac myocyte contractility in cultures and intracellular accumulation of cyclic adenosine monophosphate.[21] Cytokine imbalances may, therefore, also underlie the cardiovascular manifestations of CFS.

CFS affects women in disproportionate numbers and is often exacerbated in the premenstrual period and following physical exertion. One group[22] found that isolated peripheral blood mononuclear cells from healthy women, but not CFS patients, exhibited significant menstrual cycle-related differences in IL-1 beta secretion that were related to estradiol and progesterone levels. IL-1Ra secretion for CFS patients was twofold higher than controls during the follicular phase, but luteal-phase levels were similar between groups. In both phases of the menstrual cycle, sIL-1RII release was significantly higher for CFS patients compared to controls. The only changes that might be attributable to exertion occurred in the control subjects during the follicular phase, who exhibited an increase in IL-1 beta secretion 48 hours after the stress. These results suggest that an abnormality exists in IL-1 beta secretion in CFS patients that may be related to altered sensitivity to estradiol and progesterone. Furthermore, the increased release of IL-1Ra and sIL-1RII by cells from CFS patients is consistent with the hypothesis that CFS is associated with chronic, low-level activation of the immune system.

In contrast to the studies described above, one group[23] found no obvious difference in the levels of circulating cytokines and ex vivo production of IL-1 alpha and IL-1 receptor antagonist. Although endotoxin-stimulated ex vivo production of tumor necrosis factor-alpha and IL-1 beta was significantly lower in CFS, none of the immunologic test results correlated with fatigue severity or psychologic well-being scores. The group concluded that these immunologic tests cannot be used as diagnostic tools for individual CFS patients.

Interleukin-2 (IL-2) and soluble IL-2 receptor: IL-2, formerly termed "T-cell growth factor," is a glycosylated protein produced by T lymphocytes after mitogenic or antigenic stimulation.[1] IL-2 acts as a growth factor[2] and promotes proliferation of T cells[3] and, under particular conditions, of B cells and macrophages.[4,5]

Although serum IL-2 levels were found to be elevated in CFS patients compared with control individuals in one study,[6] decreased levels were reported in two other studies[7,8] and no difference was reported in three studies.[9-11] One group[12] reported a higher production of IL-2 by stimulated peripheral blood cells from CFS patients as compared to controls. The team who found elevated levels of IL-2 in CFS patients found no obvious relation between IL-2 serum levels and severity or duration of illness in CFS.[6]

Elevated levels of sIL-2R, a marker of lymphoid cell activation, have been found in a number of pathological conditions including viral infections, autoimmune diseases, and lymphoproliferative and hematological malignancies.[13,14] Twelve percent of CFS patients in one study[10] had elevated levels of sIL-2R, an observation that is consistent with the increased proportion of activated T cells and the reduced levels of IL-2 or decreased natural killer cell cytotoxic activity found in several studies of CFS patients. Another study found no elevation in sIL-2R levels in CFS patients.[9]

Interleukin-4 (IL-4): IL-4 acts as a growth factor for various types of lymphoid cells, including B, T, and cytotoxic T cells,[1] and has been shown to be involved in immunoglobulin isotype selection in vivo.[2] Activated T cells are the major source of IL-4 production, but mast cells can also produce it, and IL-4 has been associated with allergic and autoimmune reactions.[1] It is also noteworthy that many of the effects of IL-4 are antagonized by IFN-gamma and the decreased production of the latter may underlie a predominance of IL-4 over IFN-gamma effects. Although CD4 T cells from CFS patients produce less IFN-gamma than cells from controls, IL-4 production and cell proliferation are comparable.[3] With CD4 T cells from CFS patients (compared with cells from controls), a 10 to 20 times lower desamethasone (DEX) concentration was needed to achieve 50 percent inhibition of IL-4 production and proliferation, indicating an increased sensitivity to DEX in CFS patients. In contrast to IL-4,

IFN-gamma production in patients and controls was equally sensitive to DEX. A differential sensitivity of cytokines or CD4 T cell subsets to glucocorticoids might explain an altered immunologic function in CFS patients.[3]

Interleukin-6 (IL-6) and soluble IL-6 receptor: Most of the cell types that produce IL-6 do so in response to stimuli such as IL-1 and tumor necrosis factor, among others.[1] Excessive IL-6 production has been associated with polyclonal B-cell activation, resulting in hypergammaglobulinemia and autoantibody production.[2] As is the case with IL-4, IL-6 may contribute to activation of CD5-bearing B cells, leading to autoimmune manifestations. IL-6 also synergizes with IL-1 in inflammatory reactions and may exacerbate many of the features described for IL-1. *See* INTERLEUKIN-1 (IL-1).

The levels of spontaneously produced IL-6 by both adherent monocytes and nonadherent lymphocytes were significantly increased in CFS patients as compared to controls.[3] The abnormality of IL-6 was also observed at the mRNA level. In terms of circulating IL-6, one group[4] found that IL-6 was elevated among febrile CFS patients compared to those without this finding and therefore considered it an epiphenomenon possibly secondary to infection. Another group also found elevated levels of IL-6 in CFS patients,[5,6] but five other groups found no difference.[2,7-10]

Study of cytokine production by stimulated peripheral blood mononuclear cells from patients with a closely related syndrome to CFS, the post-Q-fever fatigue syndrome (QFS) (inappropriate fatigue, myalgia and arthralgia, night sweats, and changes in mood and sleep patterns following about 20 percent of laboratory-proven, acute primary Q fever cases) showed an accentuated release of IL-6 which was significantly in excess of medians for all four control groups (resolving QFS, acute primary Q fever without subsequent QFS, healthy Q fever vaccinees, and healthy controls). Levels of induced IL-6 significantly correlated with total symptom scores and scores for other key symptoms.[11]

CFS patients have higher levels of sIL-6R,[12] and sIL-6R enhances the effects of IL-6.

Interleukin-10 (IL-10): A study revealed that spontaneously produced levels of IL-10 by both adherent monocytes and nonadherent lymphocytes and by phytohemagglutinin (PHA)-activated nonadherent monocytes were decreased.[1] IL-10 is part of the Th2-type (humoral immunity-oriented) response.

Interstitial cystitis: Patients with CFS with chronic facial pain show a high comorbidity with other stress-associated syndromes such as interstitial cystitis. The clinical overlap between these conditions may reflect a shared underlying pathophysiologic basis involving dysregulation of the hypothalamic-pituitary-adrenal stress hormone axis in predisposed individuals.[1]

Ion channels: *See* ENERGY EXPENDITURE.

Irritable bowel syndrome: *See* GASTROINTESTINAL PATHOLOGY.

Juvenile onset chronic fatigue syndrome: *See* PEDIATRIC CHRONIC FATIGUE SYNDROME.

Lactate: *See* MUSCLE PHYSIOLOGY.

Lead poisoning: Lead poisoning can also masquerade as CFS.[1]

Learning: *See* NEUROPSYCHOLOGY.

Lentiviruses: Structures consistent in size, shape, and character with various stages of a lentivirus replicative cycle were observed by electron microscopy in 12-day peripheral-blood lymphocyte cultures from 10 of 17 CFS patients and not in controls. However, attempts to identify a lymphoid phenotype containing these structures failed and the results of reverse-transcriptase assay of culture supernatant fluids were equivocal.[1]

Light therapy: *See* SEASONAL AFFECTIVE DISORDER.

Low cysteine-glutathione syndrome: The combination of abnormally low plasma cysteine and glutamine levels, low natural killer (NK) cell activity, skeletal muscle wasting or muscle fatigue, and increased rates of urea production defines a complex of abnormalities that has been tentatively called "low CG syndrome." These symptoms are found in patients with HIV infection, cancer, major injuries, sepsis, Crohn's disease, ulcerative colitis, chronic fatigue syndrome, and to some extent in overtrained athletes. The coincidence of these symptoms in diseases of different etiological origin suggests a causal relationship. The low NK cell activity in most cases is not life-threatening, but may be disastrous in HIV infection because it may compromise the initially stable balance between the immune system and virus, and trigger disease progression. This hypothesis is supported by the coincidence observed between the decrease of CD4+ T cells and a decrease in the plasma cysteine level. In addition, recent studies revealed important clues about the role of cysteine and glutathione in the development of skeletal muscle wasting. Evidence suggests that cysteine level is regulated primarily by the normal postabsorptive skeletal muscle protein catabolism; cysteine level itself is a physiological regulator of nitrogen balance and body cell mass; cysteine-mediated regulatory circuitry is compromised in various catabolic conditions, including old age; and cysteine supplementation may be a useful therapy if combined with disease-specific treatments such as antiviral therapy in HIV infection.[1]

Lung function: *See* REGULATION OF RESPIRATION.

Lymphocytes

T Lymphocytes

CD4+ T cells (helper-inducer cells) are the principal source of "help" for antibody production by B cells in response to T-cell-dependent antigenic stimulation, as well as inducers of cytotoxic and suppressor T-cell function (CD8+ cells).[1] Discrepant results have been reported in reference to CD4+ and CD8+ cell counts in CFS patients. One group reported a statistically higher percentage of CD4+ lymphocytes with normal numbers of CD8+ cells and

CD4/CD8 ratio;[2] several groups found normal percentages of CD4+ and CD8+ cells as well as a normal CD4/CD8 ratio;[3-10] one group found decreased numbers of both CD4+ and CD8+ cells;[11] one group found reduced numbers of CD8+ cells and higher than normal CD4/CD8 ratios;[12] and one group found that most CFS subjects studied had a normal number of CD4+ cells and an elevated number of CD8+ cells that resulted in a decrease in the CD4/CD8 ratio.[13] Decreased CD4/CD8 ratios in 2 percent to 100 percent of patients have been demonstrated by other investigators.[3-6,14-16]

These conflicting results may be associated with the fluctuation in clinical manifestations of these patients or with other factors. In fact, several researchers have detected fluctuations in several immunological parameters and in the severity of symptoms in longitudinal follow-up investigations of patients with CFS. Moreover, one group found that although only marginal differences in cytokine responses and in cell surface markers were apparent in the total CFS population they studied, when the patients were subgrouped by type of disease onset (gradual or sudden) or by how well they were feeling on the day of testing, more pronounced differences were seen.[17] It is also worth noting that although one group did not find significant differences in the percentage levels of total CD3+, CD4+, CD8+, and activated, naive and memory T-cell subsets between CFS subjects and controls. They cryopreserved the cells before flow cytometric analysis and cryopreservation can differentially affect the representation of T-cell subsets.[18]

A study by one group found that elevated CD4+ and CD8+ cell counts in CFS patients were related to decreases in priming of memory, speed of memory scanning, and increases in errors on a memory fragility test.[19] However, the latter study did not control for depression severity and it is not clear whether the finding is related to comorbid depression or to CFS itself.

Although one group found a decreased proportion of CD4+CD45RA+ cells,[13] which are associated with suppressor/cytotoxic cell induction,[20] another group found no significant change in the proportions of CD4+CD45RA+ and CD4+CD45RO+ cells in CFS patients.[21] Another group also described a decrease in the number of CD4+CD45RA+ lymphocytes in two patients with severe, chronic, active Epstein-Barr virus (EBV) infection;[22] one of the two patients showed a persistent diminished number of cells despite clinical improvement with interleukin-2 (IL-2) treatment. Several publications have associated alterations in the latter subset with a number of clinical entities, particularly autoimmune diseases.[20,23-27]

Increased numbers of T cells expressing the activation marker CD26, probably as a result of CD8+ activation, have also been reported in CFS patients.[13] In this respect, an increased proportion of CD8+ cells expressing the activation marker human leukocyte antigen (HLA)-DR[8,13,28,29] have been reported in CFS patients, whereas normal proportions of CD4+ T cells co-expressing the HLA-DR marker or the IL-2 receptor (CD25) were found in one study,[8] and normal proportions of CD8+ CD38+, CD8+CD11b-, CD8+HLA-DR+ and CD8+CD28+ were found in another study,[21] and normal proportions of CD8+HLA-DR+ and CD8+CD38+ were found by another group.[30] In contrast to the latter findings, one group found significantly decreased expression of CD28 on CD8 cells[29] and three groups found significantly decreased expression of CD11b on CD8 cells.[8,28,31] Higher expression of CD38 on CD8 cells was found by three groups.[8,28,32]

It is worth noting that relatively higher proportions of HLA-DR+ T cells have been reported in a number of autoimmune disorders.[32-36] One group found that CFS patients with increased HLA-DR expression had significantly lower Short Form-36 health questionnaire (SF-36) total scores, more intense body pains, and poorer general health perception and physical functioning scores.[29] The increased expression of class II antigens and the reduced expression of the costimulatory receptor CD28, which is a marker of terminally differentiated cells, lend further support to the concept of immunoactivation of T lymphocytes in CFS and may be consistent with the notion of a viral etiopathogenesis in the illness.

Depressed responses to phytohemagglutinin (PHA) and pokeweed mitogen (PWM), an indication of dysfunction in T- and B-cell-mediated cellular immunity, were found in the CFS patients studied by most teams[3-6,13,14,17,29,37-41] while another group found no change.[17] One group found that although lymphocyte DNA synthesis in response to PHA, PWM, and concanavalin A was normal in CFS patients, the response to soluble antigens (mumps, *E. coli*) was significantly reduced.[7] Another group found that PWM-induced lymphoproliferative response is associated with Rh status among healthy controls, but not among CFS patients and the authors recommended to control future studies for Rh status.[42] In terms of the functional implications of decreased lymphoproliferative activities in CFS, one group reported that PHA-induced proliferative responses were lower in patients with poor emotional and mental health scores, and the anti-CD3/anti-CD28 response was low in those with low general health perception scores.[29] T-cell dysfunction in CFS patients has been suggested to result from decreased surface expression of CD3, an important component of the T-cell receptor complex[43] and one group found no significant increase in the mean proliferation of peripheral blood cells when stimulated with anti-CD3 antibody.[28]

B Lymphocytes

Several groups found normal levels of CD20+ resting B cells,[7-9,13,28] whereas other teams reported both increased and decreased levels.[6,10,12,16] The proportion of CD5-bearing B cells was found to be increased in two studies[10,13] or decreased in one study.[8] B cells bearing the cell marker CD5 have been associated with autoimmunity.[44]

In terms of B-cell function, spontaneous and mitogen-induced immunoglobulin synthesis is also affected as discussed later. Despite these deficits in B-cell function, stimulation with allergens provides differential lymphocyte responsiveness. Greater in vitro lymphocyte responses to specific allergens, greater baseline levels of lymphocyte incorporation of tritiated thymidine, and an increased number of immunoglobulin E-bearing B and T lymphocytes have been reported.[45,46] Elevations in the levels of certain cytokines, such as IL-4, IL-5, and IL-6 may underlie the latter effects. *See* CYTOKINES.

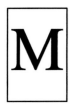

Magnesium: *See* NUTRITION.

Magnetic resonance imaging (MRI): *See* NEUROIMAGING.

Marital relationship: *See* PSYCHOSOCIAL MEASURES.

Melatonin: *See* CIRCADIAN RHYTHMS.

Memory: *See* NEUROPSYCHOLOGY.

Menstrual Cycle: *See* GYNECOLOGY.

Midodrine: *See* AUTONOMIC FUNCTION.

Mitochondria: *See* MUSCLE PHYSIOLOGY.

Moclobemide: *See* PSYCHOPATHOLOGY.

Monoamine oxidase (MAO) inhibitors: Based on the striking similarity of the clinical manifestations produced by use of the drug reserpine and the symptoms seen in patients with CFS, it was theorized that CFS was a disorder of reduced central sympathetic drive. Because of the pharmacology of control of this central sympathetic system, it was postulated that CFS symptoms would respond quickly to low dose treatment with a monamine oxidase (MAO) inhibitor. A randomized, double-blind placebo controlled study[1] using phenelzine, a nonspecific monoamine oxidase inhibitor (15 mg every other day for two weeks and then daily), in a CFS population without a diagnosis of lifetime or current psychiatric disorder or of depressed mood in the range of clinically depressed patients, showed a small but significant pattern of improvement compared to worsening in 20 self-report vehicles of CFS symptoms, illness severity, mood, or functional status. Although the data support the hypothesis of reduced sympathetic drive, an alternative hypothesis of pain alleviation is also possible. Inspired by the latter trial, a six-week trial[2] of selegeline (5 mg daily), a specific MAO B receptor inhibitor, was carried out in 25 CFS patients. Results of the trial showed a small but significant therapeutic effect in CFS (as reflected by tension/anxiety, vigor, and sexual relations variables) which appears independent of an antidepressant effect.

Monocytes: Significant monocyte dysfunction has been found in patients with CFS, such as reduced display of vimentin, phagocytosis index, and surface expression of HLA-DR.[1] These deficits respond to naloxone treatment, which suggests that increased interaction of endogenous opioids with monocyte receptors might account for the monocyte dysfunction. Another study found that although monocytes from CFS patients display an increased density of intercellular adhesion molecule (ICAM)-1 and leucocyte functional antigen (LFA)-1, they show decreased enhancing response to recombinant IFN-gamma in vitro.[2] In contrast to the latter studies, one group did not find abnormalities in superoxide anion production and phagocytosis in CFS patients.[3] Moreover, lack of a consistent elevation of neopterin, a macrophage activation marker, suggests that monocytes do not appear to account for the imbalances in IL-1 described by some groups. *See also* INTERLEUKIN-1 (IL-1) AND SOLUBLE IL-1 RECEPTORS, NEOPTERIN.

Motor function: *See* NEUROPHYSIOLOGY.

Multiple chemical sensitivity (MCS) syndrome: Multiple chemical sensitivity syndrome is part of the chemical sensitivity syndromes, which include the sick building syndrome (SBS) and the Gulf War syndrome, all related to CFS.[1,2] Except for CFS, toxic chemical exposures are accorded a significant role in their etiologies. The connections are ambiguous because of the variety of chemical agents cited and, for the most part, the relatively low levels at which exposures occur. Conventional clinical signs are also typically lacking. Explanatory mechanisms include psychiatric diagnoses such as somatization, behavioral mechanisms such as conditioning and generalization, neuropharmacological mechanisms such as sensitization (including an olfactory-limbic neural sensitization model[1] for intolerance to low-level chemicals in the environment), and psychoneuroimmunological mechanisms such as those involving the hypothalamic-pituitary-adrenal axis. Laboratory animal experimentation and controlled clinical trials, especially with inhaled material, provide the means for exploring the proffered explanations.

A study[3] of 23 patients whose sensitivities to multiple low-level chemical exposures began with a defined exposure (MCS), 13 patients with sensitivities to multiple chemicals without a clear date of onset chemical sensitivity (CS), and 18 patients meeting CDC criteria for CFS found that subjects with sensitivities to chemicals (MCS and CS) reported significantly more lifestyle changes due to chemical sensitivities and significantly more chemical substances that made them ill compared with CFS and controls. MCS, CS, and CFS patients had significantly higher rates of current psychiatric disorders than controls and reported significantly more physical symptoms with no medical explanation. Seventy-four percent of MCS and 61 percent of CFS did not qualify for any current Axis I psychiatric diagnosis. Chemically sensitive subjects without a defined date of onset (CS) had the highest rate of Axis I psychiatric disorders (69 percent). On the Minnesota Multiphasic Personality Inventory (MMPI-2), 44 percent of MCS, 42 percent of CS, 53 percent of CFS, and none of the controls achieved clinically significant elevations on scales associated with somatoform disorders. With the exception of one complex test of visual memory, no significant differences were noted among the groups on tests of neuropsychological function. Standardized measures of psychiatric and neuropsychological function did not differentiate subjects with sensitivities to chemicals from those with CFS. Subjects with sensitivities to chemicals and no clear date of onset had the highest rate of psychiatric morbidity. Standardized neuropsychological tests did not substantiate the cognitive impairment reported symptomatically. Cognitive deficits may become apparent under controlled exposure conditions.

A study[4] of 320 cases with chronic neurotoxic health impairments, of which 136 showed signs of MCS, revealed that neurotoxic substances which were used as indoor wood preservatives (mainly Pentachlorophenol and/or Lindane) were the causative agents in 63 percent of the cases with neurotoxic health impairments and MCS. Other important neurotoxic substances to which the patients were mainly exposed were organic solvents (25 percent), formaldehyde (15 percent), dental materials (15 percent), pyrethroides (13 percent), and other biocides (19 percent) (multiple exposures were possible). The time of exposure was calculated as being more or equal to ten years for 55 percent of the patients with MCS and for 50 percent of the group with neurotoxic health impairments, but without MCS. Out of the 184 cases with neurotoxic health impairments, but without MCS, there were 22 percent and, out of the 136 cases with MCS, there were 39 percent who showed all symptoms of CFS. Fifty-three percent of the cases with MCS had an allergic disposition compared to only 20 percent of the cases without MCS. In a study[5] on social support, fatigue level, being in a romantic relationship, contact with a support group on a monthly or more frequent basis, chemical avoidance in the home, gender, and an improved course of illness predicted 19 percent of the variance for perceived social support among MCS patients.

Multiple sclerosis (MS): Multiple sclerosis includes a variety of symptom complexes including paroxysmal symptoms such as trigeminal neuralgia, paroxysmal dysarthria and ataxia, parathesia and pain, paroxysmal itching, and akinesia,[1] as well as symptoms such as seizures, adventitious movements, and complications related to pregnancy and fatigue.[1] Fatigue is one of the most common findings in MS.[2-6] MS patients with progressive illness, of greater age, and those with higher Expanded Disability Status Scale scores have more fatigue.[7] This aspect is not affected by age of onset, duration of illness, gender, or index of progression. In patients with MS and in patients with CFS, subjective fatigue severity is related to impairment in daily life, low sense of control over symptoms, and strong focusing on bodily sensations.[8]

In CFS, but not in MS, there is a relationship between low levels of physical activity and attributing symptoms to a physical cause and between subjective fatigue severity and physical activity. One study[9] concluded that excessive "physiological" fatigue contributes to the symptom of fatigue in MS and is central in origin. However, since the degree of exercise-induced fatigue did not correlate with the baseline complaint of fatigue, other factors must also have been operating to produce the full range of clinical symptoms. An increase of metabolic cost of exercise did not occur in multiple sclerosis patients with mild disability, suggesting a lack or a low degree of spasticity and/or ataxia elicited by the effort. Thus, exertional capacity in MS appears to be limited mainly by poor training.[9]

Fatigue in MS is due to central, neurogenic factors and does not seem to involve any myogenic factors such as might be related to secondary muscle changes due to the long-standing disorder.[10] The subjective feeling of tiredness ("fatigue") may be related to a dissociation between central motor commands ("effort") and their mechanical consequences. One study[11] showed that acylcarnitine deficiency and fatty acid metabolic dysfunction in mitochondria were not relevant to the excessive fatigue in patients with MS. Central fatigue in

MS may also be secondary to impaired drive to the primary motor cortex and several lines of evidence strongly suggest that this is not due to a lack of motivation.[10] In this respect, one study[12] showed that pyramidal dysfunction leads to increased fatigability. Other neuroendocrine may contribute to fatigue. For instance, correlations with C-reactive protein and gadolinium-enhanced brain MRI scans suggest that activation of the hypothalamic-pituitary-adrenal axis in multiple sclerosis patients is secondary to an active inflammatory stimulus.[13] Psychological factors such as focusing on bodily sensations and low sense of control play a role in the experience of fatigue in MS and CFS.[14-17]

The treatment of multiple sclerosis encompasses two main areas: immunotherapies and management of the effects or symptoms resulting from MS.[18] It should be noted that immunotherapy with interferon-beta-1b is associated with fatigue and a study showed that only fatigue and depression were significantly associated with discontinuance of therapy.[19] Several new therapies, including tizanidine, intrathecal baclofen, botulinum toxin injections gabapentin, ondansitron, thalamic stimulation, and lamotrigine, increase our treatment options.[20] Smoked cannabis has been reported to improve (in descending rank order): spasticity, chronic pain of extremities, acute paroxysmal phenomenon, tremor, emotional dysfunction, anorexia/weight loss, fatigue states, double vision, sexual dysfunction, bowel and bladder dysfunctions, vision dimness, dysfunctions of walking and balance, and memory loss.[21] A study[22] suggests that 3,4-diaminopyridine (25 to 60 mg/day for three weeks) may play a role in the symptomatic treatment of fatigue in multiple sclerosis. However, the mechanism behind such a benefit in fatigue remains unclear and the discrepancy between subjective and more objective responses underlines the probable multifactorial nature of the pathogenesis of this symptom in multiple sclerosis. An extended outpatient rehabilitation program for persons with definite progressive MS appears to effectively reduce fatigue and the severity of other symptoms associated with MS.[23,24]

Muscle fibers: *See* MUSCLE PHYSIOLOGY.

Muscle physiology: In 21 CFS patients, the deep (muscle) versus superficial (skin, subcutis) sensitivity to pain was explored by measuring pain thresholds to electrical stimulation unilaterally in the deltoid, trapezius and quadriceps, and overlying skin and subcutis in comparison with normal subjects.[1] Thresholds in patients were normal in skin and subcutis, but significantly lower than normal (hyperalgesia) in muscles in all sites. The selective muscle hypersensitivity corresponded also to fiber abnormalities at muscle biopsy (quadriceps) performed in nine patients which were absent in normal subjects (four cases): morphostructural alterations of the sarcomere, fatty degeneration and fibrous regeneration, inversion of the cytochrome oxidase/succinate dehydrogenase ratio, pleio/polymorphism and monstruosity of mitochondria, reduction of some mitochondrial enzymatic activities, and increments of common deletion of 4,977 bp of mitochondrial DNA 150 to 3,000 times the normal values. By showing both sensory (diffuse hyperalgesia) and anatomical (degenerative picture) changes at the muscle level, the results suggested a role played by peripheral mechanisms in the genesis of CFS symptoms.[1,2]

The findings described above are underscored by a study[3] using phosphorus magnetic resonance spectroscopy on forearm muscles of ten subanaerobic threshold exercise test (SATET) positive patients (abnormal increase in plasma lactate following a short period of moderate exercise), nine SATET negative patients, and 13 sedentary volunteers. This study showed no differences in resting spectra between these groups but, at the end of exercise, intracellular pH in the SATET positive patients was significantly lower than in both the SATET negative cases and controls. The SATET positive patients also showed a significantly lower ATP synthesis rate during recovery. These observations indicate impaired mitochondrial oxidative phosphorylation in SATET positive test individuals and, since some CFS patients have a SATET positive test, they may have a peripheral component to their fatigue. In this respect, although muscle histometry (proportions of types 1 and 2 muscle fibers and muscle fiber atrophy) in CFS patients did not show the changes that would be seen as a result of inactivity (shift to predominance of type 2 muscle fibers and fiber atrophy), those patients with abnormal lactate responses to exercise (subanaerobic threshold exercise test) had a significantly lower proportion of mitochondria-rich type 1 muscle fibers.[4] Another study[5] confirmed that oxidative muscle metabolism, as measured by the maximal rate of postexercise phosphocreatine (PCr) resynthesis using the adenosine diphosphate (ADP) model, is reduced in CFS patients compared to sedentary controls and a single bout of strenuous exercise does not cause a further reduction in oxidative metabolism.

Carnitine is essential for mitochondrial energy production and orally administered L-carnitine is an effective medicine in treating the fatigue seen in a number of chronic neurologic diseases.[6,7] Amantadine is one of the most effective medicines for treating the fatigue seen in multiple sclerosis patients and isolated reports suggest that it may also be effective in treating CFS patients.[6,7] Treatment of 30 CFS patients in a crossover design comparing L-carnitine and amantadine (given for two months with a two-week washout period between medicines) showed that amantadine was poorly tolerated by the CFS patients. Only 15 were able to complete eight weeks of treatment, the others had to stop taking the medicine due to side effects. In those individuals who completed eight weeks of treatment, there was no statistically significant difference in any of the clinical parameters that were followed. However, with L-carnitine, a statistically significant clinical improvement was observed in 12 of the 18 studied parameters after eight weeks of treatment. None of the clinical parameters showed any deterioration. The greatest improvement took place between four and eight weeks of L-carnitine treatment. Only one patient was unable to complete eight weeks of treatment due to diarrhea. L-Carnitine is a safe and very well-tolerated medicine that improves the clinical status of CFS patients.[7]

Myalgic encephalomyelitis: *See* CHRONIC FATIGUE SYNDROME (CFS), DEFINITION.

Mycoplasma: Multiplex polymerase chain reaction analysis to detect the presence of *Mycoplasma genus* DNA sequences in 100 CFS patients revealed that 52 percent were infected with *Mycoplasma genus* as compared to 15 percent of healthy individuals. *Mycoplasma fermentans, hominis* and *penetrans* were detected in 32, 9 and 6 percent of the CFS patients, but only in 8, 3, and 2 percent of the healthy control subjects, respectively.[1]

Myofascial pain: *See* FIBROMYALGIA.

Natural killer (NK) cells: Natural killer cells are mostly large granular lymphocytes and constitutively cytocidal against tumor-transformed and virus-infected cells, an activity that does not require immunization.[1] Four research groups found increased numbers of NK cells,[2-5] four groups found normal numbers,[6-9] and two groups found decreased numbers of NK cells.[10,11] Despite the latter discrepancy in total numbers of NK cells measured by different groups, two groups found an increased proportion of CD56+CD3+ T cells,[12,13] which may account for the decreased NK cell cytotoxic activity seen in several studies of CFS patients, and one study found a decreased percentage of CD56+Fcgamma receptor+ NK cells, which suggests a reduced capacity for antibody-dependent cellular toxicity.[13]

Several studies revealed impaired NK cell function in CFS patients as assessed by cytotoxic activity against K562 cells.[2,6,12-19] A study on NK cell activity in a family with members who had developed CFS as adults, as compared to those who had not, documented low NK cell activity in six out of eight cases and in four out of twelve unaffected family members.[20] Two of the offspring of the CFS cases had pediatric malignancies. Based on these observations, the authors suggested that the low NK cell activity in this family may be a result of a genetically determined immunologic abnormality predisposing to CFS and cancer. Only one group[21] found elevated NK cell activity among CFS patients while another found no change.[22]

The changes in NK cell cytotoxic activity found by most groups could be related to several findings: (1) CD56+CD3- cells are the lymphoid subset with the highest NK cell activity and a decrease in their representation is expected to lower the value for the NK cell activity per effector cells; (2) the reduction in CD4+CD45+ T cells described previously may also result in decreased induction of suppressor/cytotoxic T cells; and (3) reduced NK cell activity may be associated with deficiencies in the production of IL-2 and interferon (IFN)-gamma by T cells or in the ability of NK cells to respond to these lymphokines. In terms of the latter possibility, stimulation with IL-2 failed to result in improvement of cytolytic activity in many patients with CFS.[23]

Poor NK cell function may also be related to the finding of an impaired ability of lymphocytes from CFS patients to produce IFN-gamma in response to mitogenic stimuli.[2,15] Although one study reported elevated IFN-gamma production[24] and another demonstrated normal production,[25] the inability of lymphocytes from CFS patients to produce IFN-gamma found by three groups[2,15,26] might represent a cellular exhaustion as a consequence of persistent viral stimulus. The latter postulate is supported by the finding of elevated levels of leukocyte 2'5'-oligoadenylate synthetase, an IFN-inducible enzyme, in lymphocytes of CFS patients.[18,27] Furthermore, the lack of IFN-gamma production in CFS patients may be responsible for the impaired activation of immunoregulatory circuits, which in turn facilitates the reactivation and progression of viral infections. In this respect, the IFN released as a consequence of cellular response prevents the intercellular spread of Epstein-Barr virus[28] and normal NK cell activity, but reduced EBV-specific cytotoxic T cell activity has been described in CFS patients.[29] Reactivation/replication of a latent virus (such as Epstein-Barr virus) secondary to decreased NK cell activity has also been proposed to modulate the immune system to induce CFS.[30]

More recent research has provided alternative explanations for the decreased NK cell activity observed in CFS. One study revealed a possible dysfunction in the nitric oxide (NO)-mediated NK cell activation in CFS patients based on the observations that 24 hours of treatment of NK cells with L-Arginine (L-Arg), one of the essential amino acids, enhanced NK cell activity in controls, but not CFS patients.[31] Although the expression of inducible NO synthase (iNOS) (the enzyme involved in the synthesis of NO from L-Arg) transcripts in peripheral blood mononuclear cells was not significantly different between healthy control subjects and CFS patients, and incubation with S-nitroso-N-acetyl-penicillamine, an NO donor, stimulated NK cell activity in healthy control subjects, but not in CFS patients. Addition in vitro of a glyconutrient compound (dietary supplement that supplies the crucial eight monosaccharides required for synthesis of glycoproteins) to peripheral blood cells from CFS patients significantly enhanced natural killer cell activity, increased the expression of the glycoproteins CD5, CD8, and CD11a, and decreased the percentage of apoptotic cells, parameters which were all deficient at baseline.[32] The latter observation would be consistent with a defect in glycoprotein synthesis.

In one study, 30 CFS patients were treated with IFN-alpha 2a or placebo in a double-blind crossover study.[33] Outcome was evaluated by NK cell function, lymphocyte proliferation to mitogens and soluble antigens, CD4/CD8 counts and a ten-item Quality of Life (QOL) survey. Although mean NK function rose with 12 weeks of IFN therapy, there was no significant change in the other immunologic parameters or QOL scores. When the 26 patients who completed the study were stratified according to their baseline NK cell function and lymphocyte proliferation, four groups were identified: three patients had normal NK cell function and lymphocyte proliferation when compared to normal, healthy controls, nine had isolated deficiency in lymphocyte proliferation, seven had diminished NK function only, and seven had abnormalities for both parameters. Quality of Life scores were not significantly different for the four groups at baseline. After 12 weeks of interferon therapy, QOL scores significantly improved in each of the seven patients with isolated NK cell dysfunction compared to baseline. In these patients, the mean NK cell function increased. Significant improvement was not recorded for QOL in the other three groups. Thus, therapy with IFN-alpha has a significant effect on the QOL of that subgroup of patients with CFS manifesting an isolated decrease in NK cell function.[33]

Neopterin: Neopterin is a metabolite produced during the utilization of guanosine triphosphate, and increased production of neopterin is associated with macrophage activation by interferon (IFN)-gamma.[1] Neopterin is a presumed primate homolog of nitric oxide, which activates guanylate cyclase, and is involved in neurotransmission, vasodilation, neurotoxicity, inhibition of platelet aggregation, the antiproliferative action of cytokines, and reduction of oxidative stress.[2,3] Neopterin derivatives belong to the cytotoxic arsenal of the activated human macrophage and, in high doses, enhance oxidative stress through enhancement of radical-mediated effector functions and programmed cell death by tumor necrosis factor (TNF)-alpha, while having an opposite effect at low doses.[2,4] Two groups found elevated levels of neopterin in CFS patients,[5-7] while another two found no difference with controls.[8,9] A report of nine CFS cases showed significantly elevated serum neopterin levels, in association with high Cognitive Difficulty Scale (CDS) scores,[10] and neopterin levels have been shown to correlate with levels of many other mediators that have been found to be dysregulated in CFS including members of the TNF family.[9,11,12] In terms of neurotoxicity, serum neopterin and tryptophan concentrations correlate among cancer and AIDS patients, an observation which can be accounted for by activity of indoleamine 2,3-dioxygenase, a tryptophan-degrading enzyme.[13,14] The latter enzyme also converts L-tryptophan to L-kynurenine, kynurenic acid, and quinolinic acid (QUIN). Quinolinic acid is a neurotoxic metabolite that accumulates within the central nervous system (CNS) following immune activation, and is also a sensitive marker for the presence of immune activation within the CNS.[15-17] Direct conversion of L-tryptophan into QUIN by brain tissue occurs in conditions of CNS inflammation, but not by normal brain tissue. Macrophage infiltrates, and perhaps microglia, are important sources of QUIN, an observation which is consistent with the results of inoculation of poliovirus directly into the spinal cord of rhesus macaques, resulting in increased CSF levels of both QUIN and neopterin.[15,18] Elevated serum levels of neopterin correlate with the presence of brain lesions and with neurologic and psychiatric symptoms in patients with AIDS dementia complex.[13,19] It is worth noting in this context that subcortical lesions consistent with edema and demyelination were found by magnetic resonance scans in 78 percent of CFS patients as compared to 20 percent of controls.[20]

Neurally mediated hypotension: *See* AUTONOMIC FUNCTION.

Neurasthenia: *See* CHRONIC FATIGUE SYNDROME (CFS), DEFINITION.

Neuroendocrinology: A rationale for the study of neuroendocrine correlates of CFS stems from the observation that fatigue states share many of the somatic symptom characteristics seen in recognized endocrine disorders.[1-9] Moreover, patients with CFS or fibromyalgia with chronic facial pain show a high comorbidity with other stress-associated syndromes (irritable bowel syndrome, premenstrual syndrome, and interstitial cystitis) and autoimmune conditions associated with endocrinological dysfunction. The clinical overlap between these conditions may reflect a shared underlying pathophysiologic basis involving dysregulation of the hypothalamic-pituitary-adrenal (HPA) stress hormone axis in predisposed individuals.[1-9]

Several reports have provided replicated evidence of disruptions in the integrity of the HPA axis in CFS patients. It is notable that the pattern of the alteration in the stress response apparatus is not reminiscent of the well-understood hypercortisolism of melancholic depression but, rather, suggests a sustained inactivation of central nervous system (CNS) components of this system. In this respect, one report[10] documented a significantly lower urinary free cortisol (UFC) excretion in CFS patients and a significantly higher UFC in patients with depression as compared to controls. A subgroup of CFS patients with comorbid depressive illness retained the pattern of UFC excretion of those with CFS alone, an observation that points to a different pathophysiological basis for depressive symptoms in CFS. Another study[11] further confirmed cortisol hyposecretion in saliva as well as plasma of CFS patients compared to patients with depression and controls.

Study of the detailed, pulsatile characteristics of the HPA axis in CFS patients revealed a reduction of HPA axis activity due, in part, to impaired CNS drive.[12] A diminished output of neurotrophic adrenocorticotropin hormone (ACTH), in response to administration of 100 mcg of ovine corticotropin-releasing hormone (CRH) causing a reduced adrenocortical secretory reserve that is inadequately compensated for by adrenoceptor upregulation is suggested to explain the reduced cortisol production in CFS patients.[13] Using the 1 mcg ACTH test, another study provided further evidence for a subtle pituitary-adrenal insufficiency (lower delta cortisol value) in CFS patients compared to controls.[14] Measurement of ACTH and cortisol responses following the administration of the opiate antagonist naloxone revealed that naloxone-mediated activation of the HPA axis is attenuated in CFS, an observation which renders excessive opioid inhibition of the HPA axis (an unlikely explanation for its dysregulation in this disorder).[15]

Several studies disagree with the findings described above. One study[16] found a significantly decreased diurnal change in cortisol levels, nonsignificant lower levels of morning cortisol, and higher levels of ACTH and evening cortisol among CFS patients as compared to controls. Although a relationship between adrenocortical function and disability in CFS (general health and physical functioning, functional improvement over the past year, and current social functioning) was found, no causal connection was apparent. Another study[17] failed to document a reduction in the basal activity of the HPA axis in measurements of salivary and urinary cortisol over a 24-hour period. One study[18] found slightly but significantly higher mean levels of salivary cortisol (hourly sampling over a 16-hour period) in CFS patients as compared to controls.

Other work also implicates alterations in central serotonergic tone in the overall pathophysiology of HPA axis dysregulation.[19] One study[20] found that release of ACTH (but not cortisol) in response to ipsapirone (20 mg orally) challenge was significantly blunted in patients with CFS and concluded that serotonergic activation of the HPA axis is defective in CFS.

In terms of the growth hormone/insulin-like growth factor (IGF)-1 (somatomedin C) axis, one study found that, in contrast to patients with fibromyalgia, in whom levels of somatomedin C have been found to be reduced, levels in patients with CFS were found to be elevated. Thus, despite the clinical similarities between these two conditions, they may be associated with different abnormalities of sleep and/or of the somatotropic neuroendocrine axis.[21-23] Another study[24] found attenuated basal levels of IGF-I and IGF-II in CFS patients and a reduced GH response to hypoglycemia. Insulin levels were higher and IGF-binding protein-1 (IGFBP-1) levels were lower in CFS patients compared with controls. Unlike the latter reports, no significant differences were observed among any of three patient groups (CFS, fibromyalgia, and patients with both) and controls in the mean concentration of either IGF-I or IGFBP-1 in another study.[25]

The implications of observations of neuroendocrine dysfunction is an area of intense research and interesting correlations, and therapeutic interventions are being formulated. For instance, one group[26] found that the previously described relationships in healthy women between basal circulating neutrophil numbers and plasma progesterone concentrations, and between exercise-induced neutrophilia and urinary cortisol and plasma creatine kinase concentrations, were not observed in CFS women. These observations suggest that normal endocrine influences on the circulating neutrophil pool may be disrupted in CFS patients. Moreover, the differential sensitivity of cyto-kine expression by CD4 T-cell subsets in CFS patients to glucocorti-coids might explain an altered immunologic function in CFS patients.[27]

Since both changes in endocrine and immune status variables are observed in CFS, it is noteworthy that during acute febrile illness immune-derived cytokines initiate an acute phase response, which is characterized by fever, inactivity, fatigue, anorexia, and catabolism. Profound neuroendocrine and metabolic changes also take place: acute phase proteins are produced in the liver, bone marrow function and the metabolic activity of leukocytes are greatly increased, and specific immune reactivity is suppressed. Defects in regulatory pro-cesses, which are fundamental to immune disorders and inflammato-ry diseases, may lie in the immune system, the neuroendocrine sys-tem, or both. Defects in the HPA axis have been observed in autoimmune and rheumatic diseases and chronic inflammatory dis-ease. Prolactin levels are often elevated in patients with systemic lupus erythematosus and other autoimmune diseases, whereas the bioactivity of prolactin is decreased in patients with rheumatoid ar-thritis. Levels of sex hormones and thyroid hormone are decreased during severe inflammatory disease. Defective neural regulation of inflammation likely plays a pathogenic role in allergy and asthma, in the symmetrical form of rheumatoid arthritis, and in gastrointestinal inflammatory disease.

A better understanding of neuroimmunoregulation holds the prom-ise of new approaches to the treatment of immune and inflammatory diseases with the use of hormones, neurotransmitters, neuropeptides, and drugs that modulate these regulators.[7] For instance, an article[28] proposes a possible common pathophysiology and treatment with replacement of depleted brain dopamine for post-polio fatigue and CFS based on the clinically significant deficits on neuropsychologic tests of attention, histopathologic and neuroradiologic evidence of brain lesions, impaired activation of the HPA axis, increased prolac-tin secretion, and electroencephalogram slow-wave activity seen in both conditions. Some therapeutic attempts have not yielded clearcut results, but have provided further insight into the neuroendocrinolo-gy of CFS. For instance, acute administration of the serotonin recep-tor agonist buspirone (0.5 mg/kg orally) in 11 male patients with

CFS and a group of matched healthy controls showed that CFS patients had significantly higher plasma prolactin concentrations and experienced more nausea in response to buspirone than did controls.[29] However, the growth hormone response to buspirone did not distinguish CFS patients from controls. The latter data question whether the enhancement of buspirone-induced prolactin release in CFS is a consequence of increased sensitivity of post-synaptic serotonin receptors, but open the possibility that it could reflect changes in dopamine function.[29] Although hydrocortisone treatment (13 mg/m^2 of body surface area every morning and three mg/m^2 every afternoon for 12 weeks) in a randomized, placebo-controlled, double-blind therapeutic trial was associated with some improvement in symptoms of CFS (as assessed by Wellness scale), the degree of adrenal suppression (12 out of 30 patients) precludes its practical use for CFS.[30] *See also* PSYCHONEUROIMMUNOLOGY.

Neurofeedback treatment: Electroencephalograph (EEG) neurofeedback has been identified as a potential diagnostic and treatment protocol for CFS symptoms. Test results and clinical findings of EEG neurofeedback in a CFS patient revealed improvements in cognitive abilities, functional skill level, and quality of life.[1]

Neuroimaging: Many observations suggest that CFS could derive from residual damage to the reticular activating system (RAS) of the upper brain stem and/or to its cortical projections.[1,2] It should be pointed out that, although larger right greater than left asymmetry in regional cerebral blood flow is found at the parietotemporal level in CFS patients as compared to healthy controls,[3,4] no significant correlations are found between frontal tracer uptake and right-left parietotemporal asymmetry on the one hand, and clinically relevant CFS dimensions on the other.[4] Damage to RAS could be produced by a previous viral infection, leaving functional defects unaccompanied by any gross histological changes. In animal experiments, activation of the RAS can change sleep state and activate or stimulate cortical functions. RAS lesions can produce somnolence and apathy. Studies by modern imaging techniques have not been entirely consistent,[5] but generally many magnetic resonance imaging (MRI) studies suggest that small, discrete patchy brain stem and subcortical lesions can often be seen in CFS. Regional blood flow studies by single photon-emission computed tomography (SPECT) have been more consistent.[6] They have revealed blood flow reductions in many regions, especially in the hind brain. Similar lesions have been reported after poliomyelitis and in multiple sclerosis—in both of which conditions chronic fatigue is characteristically present.[7] In the well-known post-polio fatigue syndrome, lesions predominate in the RAS of the brain stem. If similar underlying lesions in the RAS can eventually be identified in CFS, the therapeutic target for CFS would be better defined than it is at present. In this respect, [18F]fluorine-deoxyglucose (18FDG) positron emission tomography (PET) showed specific metabolism abnormalities in CFS patients (hypometabolism in right mediofrontal cortex and brainstem) as compared with both healthy controls and depressed patients.[8] The most relevant abnormality is brain stem hypometabolism, which has been also reported in single-photon emission computed tomography studies, and seems to be a marker for the in vivo diagnosis of CFS.[9,10]

Neurophysiology: A central nervous system dysfunction in CFS has been proposed based on the observation of a significant prolongation of central motor conduction time as assessed from recordings of motor evoked potentials from the Musculus Abductor Pollicis Brevis and Digiti Minimi.[1] The direct involvement of the central nervous system in the onset of CFS is underscored by the observation of gait abnormalities in CFS patients.[2] The "Prolonged Decay Test," a modified impedenzometric technique that explores any alterations of stapedial contraction, yielded significantly different clinico-audiological results in CFS patients as compared to controls and was proposed by the authors of the study as a new diagnostic test for CFS.[3] On the other hand, denervation hypersensitivity of the pupil, as a test for sympathetic oversensitivity, does not occur in CFS patients and the use of 1.0 percent topical phenylephrine had no diagnostic value in detecting CFS patients vs. normals.[4] *See also* NEUROPSYCHOLOGY.

Neuropsychology: A relationship exists between cognitive impairment and functional disability in CFS that cannot be explained entirely on the basis of psychiatric factors.[1-4] The most consistently documented neuropsychological impairments in CFS are in the areas of complex information processing speed and efficiency.[5] General intellectual abilities and higher order cognitive skills are intact, but one study[6] reported that CFS patients performed poorer on recall of verbal information across learning trials, which may be due to poor initial learning and not only to a retrieval failure. Emotional factors influence subjective report of cognitive difficulty, whereas their effect on objective performance remains uncertain. One author hypothesized that idiosyncratic cognitive processes are associated with CFS and may play a role in the maintenance of the disorder;[5] one study concluded that slowed speed of information processing and motor speed were related to low levels of physical activity;[7] and another study associated cognitive dysfunction with psychological distress in CFS.[8] Although the neuropathological processes underlying cognitive dysfunction in CFS are not yet known, preliminary evidence suggests the involvement of cerebral white matter and independence from mood disturbances.[9,10] An organic brain dysfunction, within a defined neural substrate in CFS patients, is suggested by the observation of an impaired acquisition of the eyeblink response and normal sensitivity and responsivity to acoustic or the airpuff stimuli.[11]

Although CFS and major depression and dysthymia have distinct clinical features, these disorders have slowed motor and cognitive processing speed (reaction time tasks and working memory tests) in common.[12] Nonetheless, CFS patients' ability to attend to verbal versus figural stimuli and mood ratings were different from those reported in studies of patients with depression.[13] One study found that deficits in cognitive functioning in CFS patients are more likely to be found on naturalistic than on laboratory tasks,[14] and another found that a metamemory deficit is not the cause of the memory problems reported by CFS patients.[15] At least a subset of CFS patients has a slower learning rate of verbal and visual material, and impaired delayed recall of verbal and visual information.[16,17] In one study, CFS patients were differentially impaired on the auditory relative to the visual processing task while patients with multiple sclerosis were equally impaired on both versions of the task.[18]

After physically demanding exercise, CFS subjects demonstrate impaired cognitive processing (as assessed by the Symbol Digit Modalities Test, Stroop Word Test, and Stroop Color Test) compared with healthy individuals.[19] CFS patients also show specific sensitivity to the effects of exertion at the level of effortful cognitive functioning (focused and sustained attention), which may indicate reduced working memory capacity or a greater demand to monitor cognitive processes, or both.[20,21] In CFS patients, everyday cognitive tasks may require excessive processing resources leaving patients with diminished spare attentional capacity or flexibility.[22] Self-efficacy is shown to be a significant predictor of CFS symptoms beyond the variance determined by demographic variables and distress.[23]

Neutrophils: Previously described relationships in healthy women between basal circulating neutrophil numbers and plasma progesterone concentrations, and between exercise-induced neutrophilia and urinary cortisol and plasma creatine kinase concentrations, were not observed in CFS women. These observations suggest that normal endocrine influences on the circulating neutrophil pool may be disrupted in CFS patients.[1]

Nighttime hypotension: *See* CIRCADIAN RHYTHMS.

Nitric oxide (NO): *See* NATURAL KILLER (NK) CELLS.

Nutrition: Several lines of research are being pursued concerning a possible nutritional role in the etiology or perpetuation of CFS symptomatology[1] and in this effort amino acid supplementation is an area of intense research. As discussed under Neuroendocrinology, alterations in central serotonergic tone may contribute to CFS, with one study reporting elevated levels of serotonin and another a blunted ACTH response to ipsapirone. Studies in animals and human subjects have revealed a role for the serotonergic system in fatigue after exercise and these results may be useful to understanding postexertional fatigue in CFS. Tryptophan is converted to the neurotransmitter 5-hydroxytryptamine (5-HT, serotonin) in the brain and an increase in the concentration of serotonin can result in physical and mental fatigue during prolonged exercise and can also affect sleep.[2-9] A study showed that fatigue during endurance exercise in normal individuals was increased by pharmacological augmentation of the brain serotonergic activity by serotonin reuptake inhibitors.[7] The entry of tryptophan in the brain is influenced by the plasma level of free tryptophan (that not bound to albumin) and, from competition for entry into brain, by the plasma level of branched chain amino acids. Animal studies have shown that tryptophan ingestion and the resulting raised plasma free tryptophan to competitor amino acid ratios leads to increased subjective and central fatigue. Oral administration of branched chain amino acids could prevent the increase in serotonin level during exercise and therefore delay physical and mental fatigue, but results from different reports on athletes are contradictory and the ergogenic value of amino acids needs further investigation.[7-9] Although L-glutamine was proposed to have an ergogenic effect during exercise considering its base generating potential, a study provided evidence that while low plasma and muscle glutamine concentrations may occur coincident with CFS, they may not be directly causative of fatigue or other symptoms since normalization of glutamine levels with supplementation was not associated with clinical improvement.[10] The latter results are consistent with the finding that acute ingestion of L-glutamine does not enhance either buffering potential or high intensity exercise performance in trained males.[11]

High doses of creatine supplementation improve performance during repeated sprint runs in well-trained handball players.[12,13] Further studies are needed to clarify whether low doses of creatine supplementation, after a period with supplementation of high doses, are able to maintain improved performance. Studies in CFS patients are also needed.

Low muscle glycogen levels due to consecutive days of extensive exercise have been shown to cause fatigue and thus decrements in performance. Low muscle glycogen levels could also lead to oxidation of the branched chain amino acids and central fatigue. Research on swimmers has shown that those who were nonresponsive to an increase in their training load had low levels of muscle glycogen and consumed insufficient energy and carbohydrates. However, cyclists who increased their training load for two weeks, but also increased carbohydrate intake to maintain muscle glycogen levels, still met the criteria of overreaching (short-term overtraining) and might have met the criteria for overtraining had the subjects been followed for a longer period of time. Thus, some other mechanism than reduced muscle glycogen levels must be responsible for the development and occurrence of overtraining.[14] Despite the latter results, particular forms of carbohydrate supplementation may be beneficial in CFS since addition of a glyconutrient compound (dietary supplement that supplies the crucial eight monosaccharides required for synthesis of glycoproteins) to peripheral blood cells of CFS patients in vitro significantly increased the expression of the glycoproteins CD5, CD8, and CD11a, enhanced natural killer cell activity, and decreased the percentage of apoptotic cells (all three parameters were deficient at baseline).[15]

In terms of the potential usefulness of vitamins in CFS treatment, a group[16,17] in Japan indicated that a megadose vitamin C drip infusion treatment enhanced the activity of endogenous glucocorticoids in such a way as to improve the clinical course of allergy and autoimmune disease. This group studied patients with chronic pneumonia who fit the diagnostic criteria for CFS and tested two kinds of vitamin C infusion sets, with and without concomitant oral intake of erythromycin and chloramphenicol, for treatment of the pneumonia. The dehydroepiandrosterone-annexed vitamin C infusion set (expected to enhance the endogenous activities of both glucocorticoids and gonadal steroids) was effective in patients with chronic pneumonia and CFS-like symptoms when used in combination with antibiotics while the annex-free vitamin C set was only effective in patients with the common cold.[16,17] Whether certain forms of vitamin supplementation are useful in CFS remains to be determined. One group reported ineffectiveness of high dose vitamin B-12 injections in one CFS patient.[18] Although a subset of CFS patients was reported to be folate deficient,[19] a common genetic variant affecting folate metabolism was not overrepresented in CFS[20] and a trial of liver extract-folic acid-cyanocobalamin did not yield significant effects.[21]

Electrolyte imbalances have also been proposed to play a role in CFS[22] and some scientists are investigating a possible association between ion channel abnormalities and CFS. Although chronic sleep deprivation causes a deficiency of intracellular magnesium (Mg) and decreased exercise tolerance, which can be improved by oral Mg administration,[23] one study found no association between Mg deficiency, CFS, or fibromyalgia.[24] Mg deficiency may be present in a subset of patients with spasmophilia and some groups are investigating whether Mg supplementation may benefit CFS patients.[25-27]

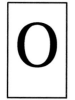

Occupational medicine: Although studies in occupational medicine have not provided evidence for an occupational etiology of CFS, they point to the relevance of distinguishing CFS from occupationally related fatigue.[1] Based on the observation that pituitary-adrenal responses to corticotropin-releasing hormone are markedly disrupted after only five days of nighttime work and that these abnormalities mimic those observed in CFS patients, one group[2] suggested that the neuroendocrine abnormalities reported to be characteristic of CFS may be merely the consequence of disrupted sleep and social routine. A Dutch study[3] found that although 23 percent of 102 veterinarians studied reported complaints of prolonged fatigue, it was likely secondary to a more than average number of daily working hours and not to allergies or exposure to infectious agents. In a sample[4] of 3,400 nurses, 202 reported six months or more of debilitating fatigue, but many sampled nurses reported a high degree of occupationally related stress, and perceived exposure to the threat of an accident as a nurse and poor physical working conditions were significantly related to symptoms reported.

Orthostatic hypotension: *See* AUTONOMIC FUNCTION.

Ovarian cysts: *See* GYNECOLOGY.

Overtraining: The overtraining syndrome, which affects mainly endurance athletes, is a condition of chronic fatigue, underperformance, and an increased vulnerability to infection leading to recurrent infections.[1,2] With a very careful exercise regimen and regeneration strategies, symptoms normally resolve in 6 to 12 weeks, but may continue much longer or recur if athletes return to hard training too soon. Psychological, endocrinogical, physiological, and immunological factors may all play a role in the failure to recover from exercise in the overtraining syndrome. One study[3] found that the parasympathetic, Addison type overtraining syndrome represents the dominant modern type of this syndrome and that functional alterations of the pituitary-adrenal axis and sympathetic system can explain persistent performance incompetence in affected athletes. Another study[4] found that overtraining does not lead to clinically relevant alterations of immunophenotypes in peripheral blood and an immunosuppressive effect could not be detected. Data from one study[5] indicated that skeletal muscle disorders may play a role in the development of symptoms experienced by the athlete with chronic fatigue, which one group termed the "fatigued athlete myopathic syndrome" and another the "Olympic fatigue syndrome".[6] *See also* NUTRITION.

Pain: No differences were found between CFS patients, major depression patients, and healthy controls for pain threshold or intolerance levels on pressure dolorimeter and ice water cold pressor tests, and neither pain threshold nor intolerance were associated with psychiatric symptoms or functional status.[1]

Parvovirus B19: The spectrum of disease caused by parvovirus B19 has been expanding in recent years because of improved and more sensitive methods of detection. Evidence suggests that chronic infection occurs in patients who are not detectably immunosuppressed. A young woman with recurrent fever and a syndrome indistinguishable from CFS was found to have persistent parvovirus B19 viremia, which was detectable by polymerase chain reaction, despite the presence of IgM and IgG antibodies to parvovirus B19.[1] Testing of samples from this patient suggested that, in some low viremic states, parvovirus B19 DNA is detectable by nested PCR in plasma, but not in serum. The patient's fever resolved with the administration of intravenous immunoglobulin.

Pediatric chronic fatigue syndrome: Although CFS was originally thought to be mainly a disease of adults, pediatric CFS is a significant problem and also the subject of much controversy.[1-10] A study encompassing chart review and telephone follow-up revealed that, although the clinical features associated with chronic fatigue in children and adolescents are similar to those described in adults, they present earlier in the course of the illness and the prognosis is better.[11] Proposed criteria for the diagnosis of CFS in adolescence are: absence of a physical explanation for the complaints, a disabling fatigue for at least six months and prolonged school absenteeism, or severe motor and social disabilities. Exclusion criterion should be a psychiatric disorder.[12] Analysis of data on severely disabled juvenile CFS patients in the United Kingdom show a modal age of onset of 11 to 15 and a tendency to deterioration in patients' cognitive and functional statuses between onset and recruitment.[13] Certain psychological factors can discriminate chronic fatigue from depressive symptomatology as well as normal functioning in children and adolescents.[14] Although an equal prevalence of CFS was found among boys and girls in two schools in England, the number of CFS cases was higher in the inner London borough-like school as compared to the more green belt borough.[15]

Personality traits: Negative perfectionism and neuroticism have been implicated as vulnerability factors in the development of chronic unexplained fatigue.[1] One author even proposes that specific somatic factors (e.g., viruses) seem to be less important for onset than certain personality traits such as depressiveness and workaholism.[2] These traits lead to an increased vulnerability to unspecific psychological or biological stressors that may cause chronic fatigue by complex psychosomatic interferences.[2] In one study, subjects with CFS, mild multiple sclerosis, and depression as well as sedentary healthy controls were administered a structured psychiatric interview to determine Axis I psychiatric disorders and two self-report instruments to assess Axis II personality disorders and the personality trait of neuroticism. The study revealed that the depressed group had significantly more personality disorders and elevated neuroticism scores compared with the other three groups. The CFS and MS subjects had intermediary personality scores that were significantly higher than healthy controls. The CFS group with concurrent depressive disorder (34 percent of the CFS group) was found to account for most of the personality pathology in the CFS sample. Another study[4] reported the finding of a mixture of neurotic and healthy defenses, and a low proportion of defenses associated with personality disorders in CFS. Psychological adaptation to CFS is similar to adaptive coping in other chronic illnesses: subjective perceptions of health status can predict functional status. Personality traits may therefore influence the perpetuation of symptomatology in CFS. *See also* PSYCHIATRIC MORBIDITY, PSYCHOPATHOLOGY.

Phosphate: Based on measurements of phosphate reabsorption by the proximal renal tubule, phosphate clearance, and renal threshold phosphate concentration, nine out of 87 CFS patients in one study[1] also fulfilled the diagnostic criteria for phosphate diabetes (phosphate depletion due to abnormal renal reabsorption of phosphate by the proximal tubule). The authors concluded that phosphate diabetes should be considered in the differential diagnosis of CFS. Further studies are needed to investigate if the possible beneficial effect of vitamin D and oral phosphate supplements should be considered in the management of CFS patients.

Phosphorus magnetic resonance spectroscopy: *See* MUSCLE PHYSIOLOGY.

Physical activity: Assessment of physical activity revealed that, although CFS patients have low activity levels similar to multiple sclerosis patients,[1-3] cognitive factors are more prominently involved in producing low activity levels in CFS than in multiple sclerosis; and in CFS, but not multiple sclerosis, a patient's activity level is related to fatigue.[1] Unlike the latter study, actigraphy in a 45-year-old CFS patient showed that measured activity was related to predictors of fatigue, but not to fatigue.[4] *See also* EXERCISE.

Platelet volume: Mean platelet volume was increased in female, but not in male CFS patients as compared to gender-matched controls.[1]

Polio vaccination: The effect of live oral poliovirus vaccination on seven CFS patients was examined in a double-blind study.[1] Vaccine administration was not associated with clinical exacerbation of CFS. However, objective responses to the vaccine revealed differences between patients and controls: increased poliovirus isolation, earlier peak proliferative responses, lower T-cell subsets on certain days postvaccination, and a trend for reduced interferon-gamma in the CFS vaccine group. Although polio vaccination was not found to be clinically contraindicated in CFS patients, there was evidence of altered immune reactivity and virus clearance.[1]

Polycystic ovarian syndrome: *See* GYNECOLOGY.

Polysomnography: *See* SLEEP.

Post-dialysis fatigue: Postdialysis fatigue has been ascribed to excessive ultrafiltration and decline in osmolality during hemodialysis but, as in CFS, somnogenic cytokines such as tumor necrosis factor (TNF)-alpha play a role.[1,2]

Post-Lyme disease syndrome (PLS): Despite antibiotic treatment, a sequel of Lyme disease may be a post-Lyme disease syndrome, which is characterized by persistent arthralgia, fatigue, and neurocognitive impairment.[1-4] Although patients with CFS and PLS share many features, including symptoms of severe fatigue and cognitive impairment, patients with PLS show greater cognitive deficits than patients with CFS compared with healthy controls. This is particularly apparent among patients with PLS without premorbid psychiatric illness.[5]

Post-polio syndrome: A possible common pathophysiology and treatment for post-polio fatigue (which affects more than 1.8 million North American polio survivors) and CFS has been proposed[1-4] based on the clinically significant fatigue, deficits on neuropsychologic tests of attention, histopathologic and neuroradiologic evidence of brain lesions, impaired activation of the hypothalamic-pituitary-adrenal axis, increased prolactin secretion, electroencephalogram slow-wave activity, and the influence of psychological factors seen in both conditions.[1,4-7] However, persistent enteroviral infection has not been consistently demonstrated in CFS. *See* ENTEROVIRUSES.

Post–Q-fever fatigue syndrome: Post-Q-fever fatigue syndrome (QFS) is characterized by inappropriate fatigue, myalgia and arthralgia, night sweats, and changes in mood and sleep patterns following about 20 percent of laboratory-proven cases of acute primary Q-fever, a condition caused by *Coxiella burnetii*[1-3] that can be transmitted through ticks, droplets, or raw milk from infected animals. This zoonotic condition is associated with high levels of interleukin-6 and, although improvement in several symptoms occurs rapidly, resolution of fatigue takes longer and it is associated with improvement in cell-mediated immunity as measured by delayed-type hypersensitivity skin responses.[3]

Postural tachycardia syndrome: *See* AUTONOMIC FUNCTION.

Premenstrual syndrome: *See* GYNECOLOGY.

Prevalence: *See* EPIDEMIOLOGY.

Progesterone: *See* GYNECOLOGY.

Prognosis: Although the prognosis of CFS is difficult to predict, cases occurring as part of clusters appear to have a better prognosis as a group than sporadic cases and those with an acute onset have a better prognosis than those with gradual onset.[1] One report[2] documented that, of 26 studies on patients with CFS or chronic fatigue, four studied fatigue in children and found that 54 to 94 percent of children recovered over follow-up periods. Another five studies operationally defined CFS in adults and found that less than 10 percent of subjects return to premorbid levels of functioning, and the majority remain significantly impaired. The remaining studies used less stringent criteria to define their cohorts. Among patients in primary care with fatigue lasting less than six months, at least 40 percent of patients improved. As the definition becomes more stringent the prognosis appears to worsen. Consistently reported risk factors for poor prognosis are older age, more chronic illness, having a comorbid psychiatric disorder, and holding a belief that the illness is due to physical causes. The latter findings were confirmed in other studies,[3,4] one of which found that the improvement rate in CFS patients with a relatively long duration of complaints is small (among 246 patients, 3 percent reported complete recovery and 17 percent reported improvement) and influenced by psychologic and cognitive factors.[3]

Prolactin: *See* NEUROENDOCRINOLOGY.

Protein kinase RNA (PKR): *See* APOPTOSIS.

Prozac: *See* SELECTIVE SEROTONIN REUPTAKE INHIBITORS (SSRIs).

Psychiatric morbidity: Since psychiatric disorders (anxiety, depression) are common in CFS and in chronic fatigue, and psychiatric status as well as physical status are associated with recovery from chronic fatigue, appropriate screening is highly relevant.[1-7] The latter statement is also valid in terms of the diagnosis of CFS. For instance, early detection of dieting disorders by adequate screening and assessment is necessary so that a significant reduction in morbidity in patients incorrectly diagnosed as CFS may occur.[8] In terms of CFS etiology, a study on patients exposed to viral meningitis showed that onset of CFS after a viral infection is predicted by psychiatric morbidity and prolonged convalescence rather than by the severity of the viral illness itself.[9] *See also* PERSONALITY TRAITS, PSYCHOPATHOLOGY.

Psychoneuroimmunology: Psychoneuroimmunology is the transdisciplinary scientific field concerned with interactions among behavior, the immune system, and the nervous system. Its clinical aspects range from an understanding of the biological mechanisms underlying the influence of psychosocial factors on onset and course of immunologically resisted and mediated diseases to an understanding of immunologically induced psychiatric symptoms. Its bioregulatory aspects include understanding the complex interaction of neuroendocrine and immunologically generated networks in maintaining health and combating disease. Psychoneuroimmunology aims at clarifying the scientific basis for humanistic medicine and at developing new models of health and illness.[1]

The nervous and immune systems respond to internal and external challenges, and communicate and regulate each other by means of shared or system-unique hormones, growth factors, neurotransmitters, and neuromodulators. Similar alterations in central catecholamine neurotransmitter levels are associated with immune activity and stressor exposure, alterations that are more pronounced in aged as opposed to younger animals.[2] For example, a decreased norepinephrine turnover in the hypothalami and brain stems of rats occurs at the peak of the immune response to sheep red blood cells,[3,4] and increased serotonin metabolism is associated with depressed Arthus reaction and plaque-forming cell response in rats stressed either by overcrowding lasting two weeks or more or by repeated immunobilization for four days.[5,6] The long-term effects of these acute changes are evidenced by chronic variable stress, which facilitates tumor growth,[7] and is associated with immune dysregulation in multiple sclerosis.[8] The hypothalamic-pituitary-adrenal axis plays a pivotal role in stress-mediated changes and stimulation of corticotropin-releasing factor in the central nervous system[9,10] has been shown to suppress rapidly a variety of immune responses, an effect which can be blocked by infusion into the brain of alpha-melanocyte-stimulating hormone (a tridecapeptide derived from pro-opiomelanocortin).[11]

Besides external stimuli, intrinsic imbalances in neurotransmitter levels affect the immune system either directly by acting on immuno-competent cells or indirectly via induction of hormonal secretions. For instance, depression is associated with neurotransmitter imbal-ances and with decreased natural killer cell cytotoxic activity.[12-15] Moreover, several studies have documented the existence of striking physiologic, neuroendocrine, metabolic, and pharmacologic differ-ences between depressed and normal subjects, and between de-pressed and severely ill subjects.[16-21]

The examples mentioned above illustrate the fact that disorders or persistent noxious stimulation of the neuroimmunological circuitry can lead to, or result from, neurological, immunological, psychiatric, or multiorgan pathology. The latter link has encouraged a search for neuroimmunological markers of CFS with functional or pathological correlates. *See also* NEUROENDOCRINOLOGY, STRESS.

Psychopathology: Several authors emphasize that somatization plays an important role in CFS both etiologically and in the perpetua-tion of symptoms,[1-8] and one study emphasizes a major contribution of avoidance behavior to functional status impairment.[9] Yet, somati-zation and illness beliefs or personality traits alone cannot explain all the experience and findings accumulated with CFS. Moreover, the diagnosis of somatization disorder is of limited use in populations in which the etiology of the illness has not been established.[10,11]

Although there is overlap between CFS and depression, and depres-sion is commonly observed in CFS,[12-14] CFS patients and those with acute infection report less severe mood disturbance than patients with depression and, in turn, patients with depression present less somatic complaints. These observations suggest that the pathophysiological processes in patients with CFS and acute infection are not simply secondary to depressed mood.[13,15] Short rapid eye movement latency has been associated with depression in the CFS population.[16] Although the studies on antidepressant therapy for CFS are affected by the different designs and methods of rating outcome, the concomitant use of other medications or therapeutic interventions, and the fact that doses of antidepressant medications administered in many studies, especially those using tricyclic antidepressants, is often much less than that normally administered in the treatment of major depressive disorder. Clinical experience dictates that antidepressant therapy is, at least, partially beneficial in CFS.[17,18] *See also* ILLNESS BELIEFS, PERSONALITY TRAITS, PSYCHIATRIC MORBIDITY.

Psychosocial measures: Some authors claim that CFS can be grouped with functional somatic syndromes, a term that refers to syndromes whose symptoms are amplified by psychosocial factors, and therefore recommend biopsychosocial intervention.[1] Psychosocial amplification is exemplified in a study[2] of 131 couples with wifes with CFS, where marital adjustment scores, wives' conflict scores, and husbands' self-empathy scores were associated with wives' CFS symptom scores. Wives with higher education, lengthier marriages, dyads with higher marital adjustment, and wives with less conflict and less support were predictive of lower problematic CFS symptoms. One study[3] investigated psychosocial morbidity, coping styles, and health locus of control in 64 cases with and without chronic fatigue identified from a cohort of primary care patients recruited six months previously with a presumed, clinically diagnosed viral illness. A significant association between chronic fatigue and psychosocial morbidity, somatic symptoms, and escape-avoidance coping styles was shown. Chronic fatigue cases were significantly more likely to have a past psychiatric history and a current psychiatric diagnosis based on a standardized clinical interview. Twenty-three of the cases fulfilled criteria for CFS. Such cases were significantly more fatigued than those not fulfilling criteria, but had little excess psychiatric disorder. A principal components analysis provided some evidence for chronic fatigue being separable from general psychosocial morbidity, but not from the tendency to have other somatic complaints. Past psychiatric history and psychological distress at the time of the viral illness were risk factors for psychiatric "caseness" six months later, while presence of fatigue, psychologizing attributional style, and sick certification were significant risk factors for CFS. Chronic illness can also be associated with a social process of marginalization that affects, for instance, employment of those affected.[4] While psychosocial factors may play a role in disease amplification, they are unlikely to account for all symptoms and changes in CFS.[5]

Psychosomatic disorders: *See* PSYCHOPATHOLOGY.

Q fever: *See* POST–Q-FEVER FATIGUE SYNDROME.

Quality of life (QOL): Quality of life is particularly and uniquely disrupted in CFS. A study[1] of 110 CFS patients revealed that overall scores on the quality of life index were significantly lower in CFS than for other chronic illness groups. Subjects reported the lowest quality of life scores in health and functioning domain. A second study[2] found that, besides physical symptoms, quality of life correlates with the hypochondriacal disposition of CFS patients toward illness.

Red blood cell distribution width: Red blood cell distribution width was increased in female, but not in male CFS patients as compared to gender-matched controls.[1]

Red blood cell mass: *See* BLOOD VOLUME.

Regulation of respiration: Because hyperventilation can produce substantial fatigue, it might be hypothesized that hyperventilation plays a causal or perpetuating role in CFS. However, in one study,[1] CFS patients and non-CFS patients known to experience hyperventilation offered substantial complaints of fatigue and hyperventilation, both to a similar degree. Hyperventilation in CFS should probably be regarded as an epiphenomenon, a conclusion that is underscored by studies that found no abnormality in the regulation of respiration in subjects with CFS.[2-4]

Rehabilitation: Seventeen out of 19 severely incapacitated CFS patients admitted to a psychiatric ward for a multidisciplinary (physical, psychological, and social) rehabilitation program showed functional improvement. This functional improvement was then maintained or exceeded by one year in 14 of these patients who were followed up.[1]

REM sleep: *See* SLEEP.

Reticular activating system: *See* NEUROIMAGING.

Rh blood group: Although pokeweed mitogen induced lymphoproliferative response was found to be associated with Rh status among healthy controls, this was not the case among CFS patients in one study.[1] The authors recommend that future studies of immunological and hematological parameters in CFS be controlled for gender and Rh status.

Rheumatoid arthritis: *See* CONNECTIVE TISSUE AND RHEUMATOLOGIC DISORDERS.

Rhinitis: *See* ALLERGIES.

RNase L: Several key components of the 2',5'-oligoadenylate (2-5A) synthetase/RNase L antiviral pathway are dysregulated in CFS.[1] A subset of individuals with CFS was identified with only one 2-5A binding protein at 37 kDa whereas, in extracts of peripheral blood mononuclear cells (PBMC) from a second subset of CFS and from healthy controls, 2-5A binding proteins were detected at 80, 42, and 37 kDa. Extracts of healthy control PBMC revealed 2-5A binding and 2-5A-dependent RNase L enzyme activity at 80 and 42 kDa. A subset of CFS PBMC contained 2-5A binding proteins with 2-5A-dependent RNase L enzyme activity at 80, 42, and 30 kDa. However, a second subset of CFS PBMC contained 2-5A binding and 2-5A-dependent RNase L enzyme activity only at 30 kDa.

Ross River virus: A prospective investigation[1] revealed that serologically proven acute infectious illness due to Ross River virus, an arbovirus most likely transmitted through mosquito bites mainly in Australia, is associated with a range of nonspecific somatic and psychological symptoms, particularly fatigue and malaise rather than anxiety and depression. Other symptoms may include headache, tenderness of the palms and the soles of the feet, arthritis, rash, and tender lymphadenopathy. Although improvement in several symptoms occurs rapidly, fatigue commonly remains a prominent complaint at four weeks. Resolution of fatigue is associated with improvement in cell-mediated immunity as measured by delayed-type hypersensitivity skin responses.

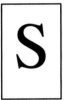 **Seasonal affective disorder:** While in one study[1] a subgroup of patients with CFS showed seasonal variation in symptoms resembling those of seasonal affective disorder, with winter exacerbation, and light therapy was suggested as a treatment alternative, another study[2] found that CFS patients exhibit an abnormally reduced seasonal variation in mood and behavior, and would not be expected to benefit from light therapy.

Selective serotonin reuptake inhibitors (SSRIs): Although antidepressant therapy is commonly used for CFS and fluoxetine (Prozac) is recommended in preference to tricyclic agents because it has fewer sedative and autonomic nervous system effects,[1] a randomized, placebo-controlled, double-blind study[2] in depressed and nondepressed CFS patients showed no significant differences between the placebo and fluoxetine (20 mg per day)-treated groups during the eight-week treatment period for any dimension of CFS (subjective assessments of fatigue, severity of depression, functional impairment, sleep disturbances, neuropsychological function, cognitions, or physical activity) in the depressed or the nondepressed subgroup. The lack of effect of fluoxetine on depressive symptoms in CFS suggests that processes underlying the presentation of depressive symptoms in CFS may differ from those in patients with major depressive disorder. A study[3] of ten male subjects without CFS revealed that fatigue during endurance exercise was increased by pharmacological augmentation of the brain's serotonergic activity by paroxetine. Therefore, SSRIs may improve the performance of CFS patients in graded exercise protocols.[4,5] Other groups propose a negative effect of serotonergic stimulation. *See also* NUTRITION.

Selegeline: *See* MONOAMINE OXIDASE (MAO) INHIBITORS.

Self-efficacy: *See* NEUROPSYCHOLOGY.

Serotonin: *See* NEUROENDOCRINOLOGY.

Sick building syndrome (SBS): Although a link has been proposed between CFS and sick building syndrome, the evidence indicates that they are distinctive entities. Sick building syndrome is an excess of work-related irritations of the skin and mucous membranes, and of symptoms such as headache (primary symptom), dry eyes, and fatigue in those working in modern air-conditioned buildings, with women reporting more symptoms than men.[1,2] One study[3] of 23 individuals concluded that the fatigue related to sick building syndrome, including CFS (15 out of 23 cases), is significantly more likely to improve than fatigue identified in sporadic cases of CFS. Chronic fatigue syndrome has no clear etiology while, besides ventilation-related problems,[4] SBS has been linked to other etiologies. For instance, in an investigation[5] of health complaints among employees of a water-damaged office building, the environment showed evidence of high-level fungal contamination with the isolation of *Stachybotrys chartarum, Penicillium, Aspergillus versicolor*, and bacteria in bulk and surface samples. A health survey of building occupants revealed a high prevalence of multiple symptoms with the predominance of neurobehavioral and upper respiratory tract complaints. The majority of symptoms were significantly less prevalent after relocation from the water-damaged environment. Exposure to toxigenic fungi may therefore be responsible for the high prevalence of reported symptoms in this group. The gap between CFS and SBS is further delineated in a case-control study[6] of over 3,300 current employees, in two state office buildings in northern California, and employees in a comparable "control" building. This study concluded that, despite the substantial number of employees with fatiguing illness in the two state office buildings, the prevalence was not significantly different than that for a comparable control building. Previously unidentified risk factors for fatigue of at least one month and at least six months identified in this population included Hispanic ethnicity, not completing college, and income below $50,000.

Silicone breast implants: Although some authors have suggested a link with CFS, immunologic sequels of silicone breast implantation such as collagen vascular diseases have not been confirmed in large studies. Nonetheless, there is a report of a 55-year-old woman who developed severe fatigue, peripheral blood eosinophilia, and hyperimmunoglobulinemia A after rupture of a silicone breast implant (SBI) during closed manual manipulation to lyse fibrotic tissue. The latter adverse effects of silicone breast implant rupture persisted over 19 years.[1] Although uncontrolled case series have reported neurologic problems believed to be associated with silicone breast implants, one review report[2] failed to find any evidence that silicone breast implants are causally related to the development of any neurologic diseases. The latter study found that although neurologic symptoms were frequently endorsed, including fatigue (82 percent), memory loss and other cognitive impairment (76 percent), and generalized myalgias (66 percent), most patients (66 percent) had normal neurological examinations. Findings reported as abnormal were mild and usually subjective, including sensory abnormalities in 23 percent, mental status abnormalities in 13 percent, and reflex changes in eight percent. No pattern of laboratory abnormalities was seen either in combination or in attempts to correlate them with the clinical situation. Laboratory studies appeared to be random without an attempt to confirm or correlate with a particular diagnosis. Diagnoses by physicians endorsing the concept that SBIs cause illness included "human adjuvant disease" in all cases, memory loss and other cognitive impairment ("silicone encephalopathy") and/or "atypical neurologic disease syndrome" in 73 percent, "atypical neurologic multiple sclerosis-like syndrome" in 8 percent, chronic inflammatory demyelinating polyneuropathy in 23 percent, and some other type of peripheral neuropathy in 18 percent. There was no coherence in making these diagnoses; the presence of any symptoms in these women was sufficient to make these diagnoses. Alternatively, after review of the data, no neurologic diagnosis could be made in 82 percent. Neurologic symptoms could be explained in some cases by depression (n=16), fibromyalgia (n=9), radiculopathy (n=7), anxiety disorders (n=4), multiple sclerosis (n=4), multifocal motor neuropathy (n=1), carpal tunnel syndrome (n=1), dermatomyositis (n=1), and other psychiatric disorders (n=3).

Sjögren's syndrome: *See* CONNECTIVE TISSUE AND RHEUMATOLOGIC DISORDERS.

Sleep: Fatigue is present in a broad range of sleep disorders and several investigators have addressed the question of whether CFS may be related to sleep disorders. In this respect, home polysomnography showed significantly higher levels of sleep disruption by both brief and longer awakenings in 18 CFS teenagers, aged 11 to 17, as compared to controls.[1] In another study,[2] CFS patients reported significantly more naps and waking by pain, a similar prevalence of difficulties in maintaining sleep, and significantly less difficulty getting off to sleep compared to depressed patients. Although sleep continuity complaints preceded fatigue in only 20 percent of CFS patients, there was a strong association between relapse and sleep disturbance. Certain types of sleep disorders were associated with increased disability or fatigue in CFS patients and disrupted sleep appeared to complicate the course of CFS. For the most part, sleep complaints in this study were either attributable to the lifestyle of CFS patients or seemed inherent to the underlying condition of CFS. They were generally unrelated to depression or anxiety in CFS. The latter conclusion stands in contrast to the finding by another group that short rapid eye movement (REM) latency is associated with depression in the CFS population.[3] Yet, another study[4] found that although the percentage of stage 4 sleep was significantly lower in 49 CFS patients, no association was found between sleep disorders and the degree of functional status impairment. Moreover, the mean REM latency and the percentage of subjects with a shortened REM latency were similar in CFS and controls. These differences in findings by different groups may be reconciled by the possibility that sleep changes are differentially distributed among subsets of CFS patients. For instance, one study[5] found that only a subgroup of CFS patients had significant daytime sleepiness and REM sleep abnormalities. Nonetheless, it should be noted that daytime sleepiness and perceived fatigue are independent phenomena and that, in one study,[6] a number of variables predicted fatigue: being female, being a smoker, high body mass index, low sleep efficiency percent, and high Minnesota Multiphasic Personality Inventory (MMPI) average clinical scale score. Fatigue should not be confused with sleepiness

and should be considered an independent symptom of sleep disturbance. Moreover, although sleep abnormalities may play a role in the
etiology of CFS, they seem unlikely to be an important cause of
daytime fatigue in the majority of patients.[7] However, pharmacological and behavioral methods that improve sleep quality may be an
important component of a pragmatically based treatment package for
patients who do have abnormal sleep.

Socioeconomic status: *See* DEMOGRAPHICS.

Sociosomatics: *See* PSYCHOSOCIAL MEASURES.

Soluble CD8 (sCD8): No elevation of sCD8 was found in CFS
patients.[1]

Soluble ICAM-1 (sICAM-1): One study found higher levels of
sICAM-1 in CFS patients,[1] an observation that is consistent with the
higher expression of intercellular adhesion molecule (ICAM)-1 in
monocytes of CFS patients.[2]

Somatization: *See* NEUROPSYCHOLOGY, PSYCHOPATHOLOGY.

Somatoform disorder: *See* NEUROPSYCHOLOGY, PSYCHOPATHOLOGY.

Somatomedin C: *See* NEUROENDOCRINOLOGY.

Spasmophilia: *See* NUTRITION.

SPECT SCAN: *See* NEUROIMAGING.

Spleen: A case report described chronic inflammatory changes of
uncertain etiology in the spleen of a CFS patient who had undergone
splenectomy secondary to trauma.[1]

Stealth viruses: *See* HERPESVIRUSES.

Stress: Based on the interrelation of the immune, endocrine, and
central nervous systems, some authors have entertained the possibility that stress and/or the reactivation/replication of a latent virus

(such as Epstein-Barr virus) could modulate the immune system to induce CFS.[1-3] For instance, patients with fibromyalgia or CFS with chronic facial pain show a high comorbidity with other stress-associated syndromes (irritable bowel syndrome, premenstrual syndrome, and interstitial cystitis). The clinical overlap between these conditions may reflect a shared underlying pathophysiologic basis involving dysregulation of the hypothalamic-pituitary-adrenal stress hormone axis in predisposed individuals.[4] Stress imposed by natural disasters such as a hurricane has also been associated with exacerbation of CFS symptoms. *See* NEUROPSYCHOLOGY, PSYCHONEUROIMMUNOLOGY.

Sub-anaerobic threshold exercise test: *See* MUSCLE PHYSIOLOGY.

Sympathetic hypersensitivity: *See* AUTONOMIC FUNCTION.

Systemic lupus erythematosus (SLE): *See* CONNECTIVE TISSUE AND RHEUMATOLOGIC DISORDERS.

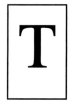 **Tapanui flu:** The 1982 publication of the resolution journal of Johann George Reinhold Forster included an account of an illness suffered by many of the sloop's crew, including Forster, after a period ashore at Queen Charlotte Sound. The symptoms of the illness were remarkably similar to those now clustered as the chronic fatigue syndrome.[1]

Temporomandibular disorders: *See* STRESS.

Testosterone: *See* ACQUIRED IMMUNODEFICIENCY SYNDROME (AIDS) AND FATIGUE.

Thyroxine: Based on the premise that individuals may experience thyroid-related symptoms such as fatigue and depression before thyroid indexes become abnormal, one exploratory, hermeneutic study described euthyroid individuals' experiences of fatigue and depression before and after low dose 1-thyroxine supplementation.[1] For women participants, the collective influence of fatigue and depression prior to treatment interfered significantly with their day-to-day lives despite their euthyroid status. For men, the influence of symptoms was far less substantial than for women. In general, participants responded favorably, both physically and emotionally, to low-dose 1-thyroxine supplementation. Furthermore, no participant experienced 1-thyroxine induced hyperthyroidism or untoward side effects attributable to 1-thyroxine. Further study of the effects of 1-thyroxine on symptoms is needed.

Transfer factors (TFs): *See* HERPESVIRUSES.

Tryptophan: *See* NUTRITION.

Tumor growth factor-beta (TGF-beta): A study found that patients with CFS had significantly higher levels of bioactive TGF-beta levels compared to healthy controls and to patients with various diseases known to be associated with immunologic abnormalities and/or pathologic fatigue: major depression, systemic lupus erythematosus, and multiple sclerosis of both the relapsing/remitting and the chronic progressive types.[1] A total of three studies supported the finding of elevated levels of TGF-beta among CFS patients.

Tumor necrosis factors (TNFs) and soluble TNF receptors: TNF-alpha and TNF-beta are cytokines produced on lymphoid cell activation.[1] Twenty-eight percent of CFS patients in one study had elevations in serum levels of TNF-alpha and TNF-beta usually with elevation in serum levels of IL-1 or sIL-2R.[2] TNF-alpha expression in CFS patients is also evident at the mRNA level, which suggests *de novo* synthesis rather than release of a preformed inducible surface TNF-alpha protein upon activation of monocytes and CD4+ T cells.[3] The levels of spontaneously (unstimulated) produced TNF-alpha by non-adherent lymphocytes were also significantly increased as compared to simultaneously studied matched controls.[4] TNF-alpha may be associated with central nervous system pathology because it has been associated with demyelination and may also lead to loss of appetite.[1,5] A study suggests that TNF-alpha may be involved in the pathogenesis of post-dialysis fatigue.[6] In contrast to the studies discussed above, one study found no difference in the levels of TNF-alpha or -beta in CFS patients[7] and two others found no differences in the levels of TNF-alpha and -beta, respectively.[8,9] The latter discrepancies are likely due to the fact that TNF levels decrease precipitously if the serum or plasma is not frozen within 30 minutes from collection.[10]

CFS patients have higher levels of sTNF-RI or sCD120a and sTNF-RII or sCD120b.[11,12] Levels of sTNF-Rs are negatively correlated with natural killer cell cytotoxic and lymphoproliferative activities in CFS, an observation that is consistent with the activities of these soluble mediators.

Tyrosine: *See* NUTRITION.

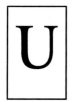

Urinary metabolites: A study of urine specimens from 20 CFS patients revealed increases in aminohydroxy-N-methylpyrrolidine (referred to as chronic fatigue symptom urinary marker 1, or CFSUM1), tyrosine, beta-alanine, aconitic acid, and succinic acid and reductions in an unidentified urinary metabolite, CFSUM2, alanine, and glutamic acid. CFSUM1, beta-alanine, and CFSUM2 were found by discriminant function analysis to be the first, second, and third most important metabolites, respectively, for discriminating between CFS and non-CFS subjects. The abundances of CFSUM1 and beta-alanine were positively correlated with symptom incidence, symptom severity, core CFS symptoms, and symptom core list (SCL)-90-R somatization, suggesting a molecular basis for CFS.[1] In a second report by the same group, severe fatigue was the only symptom with 100 percent sensitivity and specificity and CFSUM1 excretion was the primary metabolite for expression of this symptom. All symptom indices analyzed (symptom indices of total symptom incidence, CFS core symptoms, cognitive, neurological, musculoskeletal, gastrointestinal, infection-related and genitourinary symptom indices, as well as a visual analogue pain scale of average pain intensity) had elevated responses in the CFS patients and significant correlations with changes in the urinary excretion of metabolites. CFSUM1 and beta-alanine were the first and second metabolites correlated with the CFS core symptom index and CFSUM1 was primarily associated with infection-related and musculoskeletal indexes whereas beta-alanine was primarily associated with gastrointestinal and genitourinary indexes.[2]

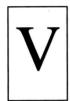

Vitamins: *See* NUTRITION.

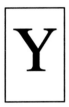

Yersinia: A study based on the detection of antibodies to various *Yersinia* outer membrane proteins (YOPs) in serum samples from 88 CFS patients and 77 healthy age- and gender-matched controls concluded that *Yersinia enterocolitica* is unlikely to play a major role in the etiology of CFS.[1]

Notes

Acquired immunodeficiency syndrome (AIDS) and fatigue

1. Rose L, Pugh LC, Lears K, Gordon DL. The fatigue experience: Persons with HIV infection. *Journal of Advanced Nursing* 28(2):295-304, 1998.

2. Soucy MD. Fatigue and depression: Assessment in human immunodeficiency virus disease. *Nurse Practitioner Forum* 8(3):121-125, 1997.

3. Breitbart W, McDonald MV, Rosenfeld B, Monkman ND, Passik S. Fatigue in ambulatory AIDS patients. *Journal of Pain & Symptom Management* 15(3):159-167, 1998.

4. Walker K, McGown A, Jantos M, Anson J. Fatigue, depression, and quality of life in HIV-positive men. *Journal of Psychosocial Nursing & Mental Health Services* 35(9):32-40, 1997.

5. Grady C, Anderson R, Chase GA. Fatigue in HIV-infected men receiving investigational interleukin-2. *Nursing Research* 47(4):227-234, 1998.

6. Darko DF, Mitler MM, Miller JC. Growth hormone, fatigue, poor sleep, and disability in HIV infection. *Neuroendocrinology* 67(5):317-324, 1998.

7. Wagner GJ, Rabkin JG, Rabkin R. Testosterone as a treatment for fatigue in HIV+ men. *General Hospital Psychiatry* 20(4):209-213, 1998.

8. Wagner GJ, Rabkin JG. Testosterone, illness progression, and megestrol use in HIV-positive men. *Journal of AIDS & Human Retrovirology* 17(2):179-180, 1998.

Allergies

1. Conti F, Magrini L, Priori R, Valesini G, Bonini S. Eosinophil cationic protein serum levels and allergy in chronic fatigue syndrome. *Allergy* 51(2):124-127, 1992.

2. Steinberg P, Pheley A, Peterson PK. Influence of immediate hypersensitivity skin reactions on delayed reactions in patients with chronic fatigue syndrome. *Journal of Allergy & Clinical Immunology* 98(6 Pt 1):1126-1128, 1996.

3. Baraniuk JN, Clauw D, MacDowell-Carneiro AL, Bellanti J, Pandiri P, Foong S, Ali M. IgE concentrations in chronic fatigue syndrome. *Journal of Chronic Fatigue Syndrome* 4(1):13-22, 1998.

4. Lloyd AR, Wakefield D, Boughton CR et al. Immunological abnormalities in the chronic fatigue syndrome. *Medical Journal of Australia* 151:122-124, 1989.

5. Lloyd A, Hickie I, Hickie C, Dwyer J, Wakefield D. Cell-mediated immunity in patients with chronic fatigue syndrome, healthy controls and patients with major depression. *Clinical and experimental Immunology* 87(1):76-79, 1992.

6. Steinberg P, McNutt BE, Marshall P, Schenck C, Lurie N, Pheley A, Peterson PK. Double-blind placebo-controlled study of the efficacy of oral terfenadine in the treatment of chronic fatigue syndrome. *Journal of Allergy & Clinical Immunology* 97(1 Pt 1):119-126, 1996.

7. Mawle AC, Nisenbaum R, Dobbins JG, Gary HE Jr, Stewart JA, Reyes M, Steele L, Schmid DS, Reeves WC. Immune responses associated with chronic fatigue syndrome: A case-control study. *The Journal of Infectious Diseases* 175(1): 136-141, 1997.

8. Baraniuk JN, Clauw DJ, Gaumond E. Rhinitis symptoms in chronic fatigue syndrome. *Annals of Allergy, Asthma, & Immunology* 81(4):359-365, 1998.

9. Borish L, Schmaling K, DiClementi JD, Streib J, Negri J, Jones JF. Chronic fatigue syndrome: Identification of distinct subgroups on the basis of allergy and psychologic variables. *Journal of Allergy & Clinical Immunology* 102(2):222-230, 1998.

10. Borok G. Chronic fatigue syndrome: an atopic state. *Journal of Chronic Fatigue Syndrome* 4(3):39-58, 1998.

Antidiuretic hormone (ADH)/Arginine vasopressin

1. Peroutka SJ. Chronic fatigue disorders: an inappropriate response to arginine vasopressin? *Medical Hypotheses* 50(6):521-523, 1998.

2. De Lorenzo F, Hargreaves J, Kakkar VV. Pathogenesis and management of delayed orthostatic hypotension in patients with chronic fatigue syndrome. *Clinical Autonomic Research* 7(4):185-190, 1997.

Apoptosis

1. Hassan IS, Bannister BA, Akbar A, Weir W, Bofill M. A study of the immunology of the chronic fatigue syndrome: Correlation of immunologic markers to health dysfunction. *Clinical Immunology & Immunopathology* 87(1):60-67, 1998.

2. Vojdani A, Ghoneum M, Choppa PC, Magtoto L, Lapp CW. Elevated apoptotic cell population in patients with chronic fatigue syndrome: The pivotal role of protein kinase RNA. *Journal of Internal Medicine* 242(6):465-478, 1997.

3. See DM, Cimoch P, Chou S, Chang J, Tilles J. The in vitro immunodulatory effects of glyconutrients on peripheral blood mononuclear cells of patients with chronic fatigue syndrome. *Integrative Physiological & Behavioral Science* 33(3): 280-287, 1998.

4. Swanink CM, Vercoulen JH, Galama JM, Roos MT, Meyaard L, van der Ven-Jongekrijg J, de Nijs R, Bleijenberg G, Fennis JF, Miedema F, van der Meer JW. Lymphocyte subsets, apoptosis, and cytokines in patients with chronic fatigue syndrome. *The Journal of Infectious Diseases* 173(2):460-463, 1996.

Autoimmunity

1. Konstantinov K, von Mikecz A, Buchwald D, Jones J, Gerace L, Tan EM. Autoantibodies to nuclear antigens in chronic fatigue syndrome. *Journal of Clinical Investigation* 98(8):1888-1896, 1996.

2. Poteliakhoff A. Fatigue syndromes and the aetiology of autoimmune disease. *Journal of Chronic Fatigue Syndrome* 4(4):31-50 1998.

3. von Mikecz A, Konstantinov K, Buchwald DS, Gerace L, Tan EM. High frequency of autoantibodies in patients with chronic fatigue syndrome. *Arthritis & Rheumatism* 40(2):295-305, 1997.

4. Keller RH, Lane JL, Klimas N, Reiter WM, Fletcher MA, van Riel F, Morgan R. Association between HLA class II antigens and the chronic fatigue immune dysfunction syndrome. *Clinical Infectious Diseases* 18(Suppl 1):S154-S156, 1994.

5. Jones J. Serologic and immunologic responses in chronic fatigue syndrome with emphasis on the Epstein-Barr virus. *Reviews of Infectious Diseases* 13(1): S26-S31, 1991.

6. Jones JF, Straus SE. Chronic Epstein-Barr virus infection. *Annual Revue of Medicine* 38:195-209, 1987.

7. Jones JF, Ray G, Minnich LL et al. Evidence for active Epstein-Barr virus infection in patients with persistent, unexplained illnesses: elevated anti-early antigen antibodies. *Annals of Internal Medicine* 102:1-7, 1985.

8. Kaslow JE, Rucker L, Onishi R. Liver extract-folic acid-cyanocobalamin vs. placebo for chronic fatigue syndrome. *Archives of Internal Medicine* 149:2501-2503, 1989.

9. Prieto J, Subira ML, Castilla A et al. Naloxone-reversible monocyte dysfunction in patients with chronic fatigue syndrome. *Scandinavian Journal of Immunology* 30:13-20, 1989.

10. Salit IE. Sporadic postinfectious neuromyasthenia. *Canadian Medical Association Journal* 133:659-663, 1985.

11. Straus SE, Tosato G, Armstrong G et al. Persisting illness and fatigue in adults with evdience of Epstein-Barr virus infection. *Annals of Internal Medicine* 102:7-16, 1985.

12. Tobi M, Morag A, Ravid Z et al. Prolonged atypical illness associated with serological evidence of persistent Epstein-Barr infection. *Lancet* 1:61-64, 1982.

13. Bates DW, Buchwald D, Lee J, Kith P, Doolittle T, Rutherford C, Churchill WH, Schur PH, Werner M, Wybenga D et al. Clinical laboratory test findings in patients with chronic fatigue syndrome. *Archives of Internal Medicine* 155:97-103, 1995.

14. Gold D, Bowden R, Sixbey J et al. Chronic fatigue. A prospective clinical and virologic study. *JAMA* 264:48-53, 1990.

15. Behan PO, Behan WHM, Bell EJ. The postviral fatigue syndrome—An analysis of the findings in 50 cases. *Journal of Infection* 10:211-222, 1985.

16. Weinstein L. Thyroiditis and "chronic infectious mononucleosis." *New England Journal of Medicine* 317:1225-1226, 1987.

17. Plioplys AV. Antimuscle and anti-CNS circulating antibodies in chronic fatigue syndrome. *Neurology* 48(6):1717-1719, 1997.

18. Rasmussen AK, Nielsen AH, Andersen V, Barington T, Bendtzen K, Hansen MB, Nielsen L, Pederson BK, Wiik A. Chronic fatigue syndrome—a controlled cross sectional study. *The Journal of Rheumatology* 21(8):1527-1531, 1994.

19. Itoh Y, Hamada H, Imai T, Saki T, Igarashi T, Yuge K, Fukunaga Y, Yamamoto M. Antinuclear antibodies in children with chronic nonspecific complaints. *Autoimmunity* 25(4):243-250, 1997.

Autonomic function

1. Rowe PC, Calkins H. Neurally mediated hypotension and chronic fatigue syndrome. *American Journal of Medicine* 105(3A):15S-21S, 1998.

2. Streeten DH, Anderson GH Jr. The role of delayed orthostatic hypotension in the pathogenesis of chronic fatigue syndrome. *Clinical Autonomic Research* 8(2):119-124, 1998.

3. Freeman R, Komaroff AL. Does the chronic fatigue syndrome involve the autonomic nervous system? *American Journal of Medicine* 102(4):357-364, 1997.

4. De Lorenzo F, Hargreaves J, Kakkar VV. Possible relationship between chronic fatigue and postural tachycardia syndromes. *Clinical Autonomic Research* 6(5):263-264, 1996.

5. De Lorenzo F, Kakkar VV. Twenty-four-hour urine analysis in patients with orthostatic hypotension and chronic fatigue syndrome. *Australian & New Zealand Journal of Medicine* 26(6):849-850, 1996.

6. De Lorenzo F, Hargreaves J, Kakkar VV. Pathogenesis and management of delayed orthostatic hypotension in patients with chronic fatigue syndrome. *Clinical Autonomic Research* 7(4):185-190, 1997.

7. Klonoff DC. Chronic fatigue syndrome and neurally mediated hypotension. *JAMA* 275(5):359-360, 1996.

8. Wilke WS, Fouad-Tarazi FM, Cash JM, Calabrese LH. The connection between chronic fatigue syndrome and neurally mediated hypotension. *Cleveland Clinical Journal of Medicine* 65(5):261-266, 1998.

9. Chester AC. Neurally mediated hypotension, chronic fatigue syndrome and upper aerodigestive tract reflexes. *Integrative Physiological & Behavioral Science* 32(2):160-161, 1997.

10. Stewart J, Weldon A, Arlievsky N, Li K, Munoz J. Neurally mediated hypotension and autonomic dysfunction measured by heart rate variability during head-up tilt testing in children with chronic fatigue syndrome. *Clinical Autonomic Research* 8(4):221-230, 1998.

11. Baschetti R. Chronic fatigue syndrome and neurally mediated hypotension. *JAMA* 275(5):359; discussion 360, 1996.

12. Beard TC. Chronic fatigue syndrome and neurally mediated hypotension. *JAMA* 275(5):359; discussion 360, 1996.

13. Lehmann M, Foster C, Dickhuth HH, Gastmann U. Autonomic imbalance hypothesis and overtraining syndrome. *Medicine & Science in Sports & Exercise* 30(7):1140-1145, 1998.

14. Cordero DL, Sisto SA, Tapp WN, LaManca JJ, Pareja JG, Natelson BH. Decreased vagal power during treadmill walking in patients with chronic fatigue syndrome. *Clinical Autonomic Research* 6(6):329-333, 1996.

15. Nozawa I, Imamura S, Fujimori I, Hashimoto K, Nakayama H, Hisamatsu K, Murakami Y. The relationship between psychosomatic factors and orthostatic

dysregulation in young men. *Clinical Otolaryngology & Allied Sciences* 22(2):135-138, 1997.

16. De Becker P, Dendale P, De Meirleir K, Campine I, Vandenborne K, Hagers Y. Autonomic testing in patients with chronic fatigue syndrome. *American Journal of Medicine* 105(3A):22S-26S, 1998.

17. Yataco A, Talo H, Rowe P, Kass DA, Berger D, Calkins H. Comparison of heart rate variability in patients with chronic fatigue syndrome and controls. *Clinical Autonomic Research* 7(6):293-297, 1997.

18. Smit AA, Bolweg NM, Lenders JW, Wieling W. No strong evidence of disturbed regulation of blood pressure in chronic fatigue syndrome. *Nederlands Tijdschrift voor Geneeskunde* 142(12):625-658, 1998.

19. Duprez DA, De Buyzere ML, Drieghe B, Vanhaverbeke F, Taes Y, Michielsen W, Clement DL. Long- and short-term blood pressure and RR-interval variability and psychosomatic distress in chronic fatigue. *Clinical Science* 94(1):57-63, 1998.

20. Sendrowski DP, Buker EA, Gee SS. An investigation of sympathetic hypersensitivity in chronic fatigue syndrome. *Optometry & Vision Science* 74(8):660-663, 1997.

21. Cruz DN, Mahnensmith RL, Perazella MA. Intradialytic hypotension: Is midodrine beneficial in symptomatic hemodialysis patients? *American Journal of Kidney Disease* 30(6):772-779, 1997.

22. Handa KK, Sra JS, Akhtar M. Successful treatment of a patient with chronic fatigue using head-up tilt guided therapy. *Wisconsin Medical Journal* 96(3):40-42, 1997.

Beta-2 microglobulin

1. Buchwald D, Wener MH, Pearlman T, Kith P. Markers of inflammation and immune activation in chronic fatigue and chronic fatigue syndrome. *The Journal of Rheumatology* 24(2):372-376, 1997.

2. Patarca R, Klimas NG, Garcia MN, Pons H, Fletcher MA. Dysregulated expression of soluble immune mediator receptors in a subset of patients with chronic fatigue syndrome: Categorization of patients by immune status. *Journal of Chronic Fatigue Syndrome* 1:79-94, 1995.

3. Patarca R, Klimas NG, Sandler D, Garcia MN, Fletcher MA. Interindividual immune status variation patterns in patients with chronic fatigue syndrome: association with the tumor necrosis factor system and gender. *Journal of Chronic Fatigue Syndrome* 2(1):13-19, 1995.

4. Chao CC, Gallagher M, Phair J, Peterson PK. Serum neopterin and interleukin-6 levels in chronic fatigue syndrome. *The Journal of Infectious Diseases* 162:1412-1413, 1990.

Blood volume

1. Streeten DHP, Bell DS. Circulating blood volume in chronic fatigue syndrome. *Journal of Chronic Fatigue Syndrome* 4(1):3-12, 1998.

2. Jelkmann W, Wolff M, Fandrey J. Modulation of the production of erythropoietin by cytokines: In vitro studies and their clinical implications. *Eryhtropoeitin in the 90s.* Schaefer RM, Heidland A, Hörl WH (eds.), Contributions in Nephology. Basel, Karger, 1990, Germany, 1995, Vol 87, pp. 68-77.

3. Patarca R, Lugtendorf S, Antoni M, Klimas NG, Fletcher MA. Dysregulated expression of tumor necrosis factor in the chronic fatigue immune dysfunction syndrome: Interrelations with cellular sources and patterns of soluble immune mediator expression. *Clinical Infectious Diseases* 18:S147-S153, 1994.

Borna disease virus (BDV)

1. Nakaya T, Kuratsune H, Kitani T, Ikuta K. Demonstration on borna disease virus in patients with chronic fatigue syndrome. *Nippon Rinsho—Japanese Journal of Clinical Medicine* 55(11):3064-3071, 1997.

2. Kitani T, Kuratsune H, Fuke I, Nakamura Y, Nakaya T, Asahi S, Tobiume M, Yamaguti M, Machii T, Inagi R, Yamanishi K, Ikuta K. Possible correlation between borna disease virus infection and Japanese patients with chronic fatigue syndrome. *Microbiology & Immunology* 40(6):459-462, 1996.

3. Nakaya T, Takahashi H, Nakamura Y, Asahi S, Tobiume M, Kuratsune H, Kitani T, Yamanishi K, Ikuta K. Demonstration of borna disease virus RNA in peripheral blood mononuclear cells derived from Japanese patients with chronic fatigue syndrome. *FEBS Letters* 378(2):145-149, 1996.

Brain injury and fatigue

1. LaChapelle DL, Finlayson MA. Brain injury and healthy controls. *Brain Injury* 12(8):649-659, 1998.

Cancer and fatigue

1. Levine PH, Fears TR, Cummings P, Hoover RN. An evaluation of subjective and objective measures of fatigue in patients with cancer and a fatiguing illness in Northern Nevada. *Annals of Epidemiology* 8(4):245-249, 1998.

2. Stone P, Richards M, Hardy J. Fatigue in patients with cancer. *European Journal of Cancer Care* 34(11):1670-1676, 1998.

3. Mock V. Breast cancer and fatigue: Issues for the workplace. *AAOHN Journal* 46(9):425-431, 1998.

4. Vastag B, Beidler N. Tired out: Patients find easy answers for cancer-related fatigue. *Journal of the National Cancer Institute* 90(21):1591-1594, 1998.

5. Schneider RA. Concurrent validity of the Beck depression inventory and the multidimensional fatigue inventory-20 in assessing fatigue among cancer patients. *Psychological Reports* 82(3 Pt 1):883-886, 1998.

6. Yarbro CH. Intervention for fatigue. *European Journal of Cancer Care (English Language Edition)* 5(2 Suppl):35-38, 1996.

7. Labots E, Puhlmann G. Report action on fatigue and its consequences. *Oncologica* 14(2):29-32, 1997.

8. Alberts M, Smets EM, Vercoulen JH, Garssen B, Bleijenberg G. "Abbreviated fatigue questionnaire": A practical tool in the classification of fatigue. *Nederlands Tijdschrift voor Geneeskunde* 141(31):1526-1530, 1997.

9. Hockenberry-Eaton M, Hinds, PS, Alcoser, P, O'Neill, JB, Euell, K, Howard, V, Gattuso, J, Taylor, J. Fatigue in children and adolescents with cancer. *Journal of Pediatric Oncology Nursing* 15(3):172-182, 1998.

10. Stein KD, Martin SC, Hann DM, Jacobsen PB. A multidimensional measure of fatigue for use with cancer patients. *Cancer Practice* 6(3):143-152, 1998.

11. Schneider RA. Reliability and validity of the multidimensional fatigue inventory (MFI-20) and the Rhoten fatigue scale among rural cancer outpatients. *Cancer Nursing* 21(5):370-373, 1998.

12. Newell S, Sanson-Fisher RW, Girgis A, Bonaventura A. How well do medical oncologists' perceptions reflect their patients' reported physical and psychosocial problems? Data from a survey of five oncologists. *Cancer* 83(8):1640-1651, 1998.

13. Pater JL, Zee B, Palmer M, Johnston D, Osoba D. Fatigue in patients with cancer: Results with National Cancer Institute of Canada clinical trials group studies employing the EORTC QLQ-C30. *Supportive Care in Cancer* 5(5):410-413, 1997.

14. Smets EM, Visser MR, Garssen B, Frijda NH, Oosterveld P, de Haes JC. Understanding the level of fatigue in cancer patients undergoing radiotherapy. *Journal of Psychosomatic Research* 45(3):277-293, 1998.

15. Smets EM, Visser MR, Willems-Groot AF, Garssen B, Oldenburger F, van Tienhoven G, de Haes JC. Fatigue and radiotherapy: (a) experience in patients undergoing treatment. *British Journal of Cancer* 78(7):899-906, 1998.

16. Smets EM, Visser MR, Willems-Groot AF, Garssen B, Schuster-Uitterhoeve AL, de Haes JC. Fatigue and radiotherapy: (b) experience in patients nine months following treatment. *British Journal of Cancer* 78(7):907-912, 1998.

17. Woo B, Dibble SL, Piper BF, Keating SB, Weiss MC. Differences in fatigue by treatment methods in women with breast cancer. *Oncology Nursing Forum* 25(5):915-920, 1998.

18. Dimeo F, Rumberger BG, Keul J. Aerobic exercise as therapy for cancer fatigue. *Medicine & Science in Sports & Exercise* 30(4):475-478, 1998.

Cardiovascular deconditioning

1. De Lorenzo F, Xiao H, Mukherjee M, Harcup J, Suleiman S, Kadziola Z, Kakkar VV. Chronic fatigue syndrome: Physical and cardiovascular deconditioning *Quarterly Journal of Medicine* 91(7):475-481, 1998.

2. Rowbottom D, Keast D, Pervan Z, Morton A. The physiological response to exercise in chronic fatigue syndrome. *Journal of Chronic Fatigue Syndrome* 4(2):33-50, 1998.

Chlorinated hydrocarbons

1. Dunstan RH, Roberts TK, Donohoe M, McGregor NR, Hope D, Taylor WG, Watkins JA, Murdoch RN, Butt HL. Bioaccumulated chlorinated hydrocarbons and red/white blood cell parameters. *Biochemical and Molecular Medicine* 58(1):77-84, 1996.

2. Dunstan RH, Donohoe M, Taylor W, Roberts TK, Murdoch RN, Watkins JA, McGregor NR. Chlorinated hydrocarbons and chronic fatigue syndrome. *Medical Journal of Australia* 164(4):251, 1996.

Chronic fatigue syndrome (CFS), definition

1. Chronic fatigue syndrome. Baschetti R. *JAMA* 279(6):431-433, 1998; *Quarterly Journal of Medicine* 90(11):723, 1997; Chester AC. *JAMA* 279(6):432-3, 1998; Czarnowski D, Panasiuk B, Wiercinska-Drapalo A, Puzanowska B, Prokopowicz D. *Polskie Archiwum Medycyny Wewnetrznej* 96(2):161-164, 1996; David A, Wessely S. *Lancet* 348(9038):1385, 1996; Demitrack MA, Engleberg NC. *Current Therapy in Endocrinology & Metabolism* 6:152-160, 1997; Devitt NF. *JAMA* 279(6):432; discussion 432-433, 1997; Egyedi P. *Nederlands Tijdschrift voor Geneeskunde* 141(37):1790-1791, 1997; Fisher L. *Professional Nurse* 12(8):578-581, 1997; Hedrick TE. *Quarterly Journal of Medicine* 90(11):723-725, 1997; Knepper S. *Nederlands Tijdschrift voor Geneeskunde* 141(48):2360, 1997; Kendell R, Turnberg L, Toby J. *Lancet* 348(9038):1384, 1996; Koehoorn J, Fechter MM, de Vries H. *Nederlands Tijdschrift voor Geneeskunde* 141(48):2362-2363, 1997; Kroneman H, Croon NH. *Nederlands Tijdschrift voor Geneeskunde* 141(37):1791, 1997; Litzman J, Lokaj J, Fucikova T. *Casopis Lekaru Ceskych* 137(10):295-298, 1998; Loblay RH. *Lancet* 351(9111):1292, 1998; Mawle AC. *Immunological Investigations* 26(1-2):269-273, 1997; Mayou R. *Lancet* 348(9038):1384-1385, 1996; Rouillon F, Delhommeau L, Vinceneux P. *Presse Medicale* 25(40):2031-2036, 1996; Sharpe M. *Psychiatric Clinics of North America* 19(3):549-573, 1996; Shepherd C. *Professional Nurse* 12(11):827, 1997; Shepherd C. *Lancet* 349(9044):57-58, 1997; Smits MG, Nagtegaal JE, Swart AC. *Nederlands Tijdschrift voor Geneeskunde* 141(48):2359-2360, 1997; Sobetzko HM, Stark FM. *Nervenarzt* 68(11):924-925, 1997; Straus SE *British Medical Journal* 313(7061):831-832, 1996; Studd J, Panay N. *Lancet* 348(9038):1384, 1996; Sykes R. *British Journal of Psychiatry* 171:393, 1997; van der Meer JW. *Nederlands Tijdschrift voor Geneeskunde* 141(31): 1507-1509, 1997; van der Meer JW. *European Journal of Clinical Investigation* 27(4):255-256, 1997; Van Dishoeck EA. *Nederlands Tijdschrift voor Geneeskunde* 141(48):2358-2359, 1997; Van Houdenhove B, Fischler B, Neerinckx E. *Nederlands Tijdschrift voor Geneeskunde* 141(48):2360-2361, 1997; Vooren PH. *Nederlands Tijdschrift voor Geneeskunde* 141(48):2359, 1997; Wijlhuizen T, Hamerslag M. *Nederlands Tijdschrift voor Geneeskunde* 141(48):2361-2362, 1997.

2. Wessely S. Chronic fatigue syndrome: A 20th century illness? *Scandinavian Journal of Work, Environment & Health* 23 (Suppl 3):17-34, 1997. Layzer RB. Asthenia and the chronic fatigue syndrome. *Muscle & Nerve* 21(12):1609-1611, 1998.

3. Cheung F, Lin KM. Neurasthenia, depression and somatoform disorder in a Chinese-Vietnamese woman migrant. *Culture, Medicine & Psychiatry* 1997; 21(2): 247-58.

4. Hickie I, Hadzi-Pavlovic D, Ricci C. Reviving the diagnosis of neurasthenia. *Psychological medicineicine* 27(5):989-994, 1997.

5. Massey RU. Neurasthenia, psychasthenia, CFS, and related mattters. *Connecticut Medicine* 60(10):627-628, 1996.

6. Clauw DJ, Chrousos GP. Chronic pain and fatigue syndromes: Overlapping clinical and neuroendocrine features and potential pathogenic mechanisms. *Neuroimmunomodulation* 4(3):134-153, 1997.

7. van der Meer JW, Elving LD. Chronic fatigue—"cured with 23 I's." *Nederlands Tijdschrift voor Geneeskunde* 141(31):1505-1507, 1997.

8. van der Meer JW, Rijken PM, Bleijenberg G, Thomas S, Hinloopen RJ, Bensing JM. Indications for management in long-term, physically unexplained fatigue symptoms. *Nederlands Tijdschrift voor Geneeskunde* 141(31):1516-1519, 1997.

9. Wessely S. The epidemiology of chronic fatigue syndrome. *Epidemiologia E Psichiatria Sociale* 7(1):10-24, 1998.

10. Levine PH. Chronic fatigue syndrome comes of age. *American Journal of Medicine* 105(3A):2S-6S, 1998.

11. Lee P. Recent developments in chronic fatigue syndrome. *American Journal of Medicine* 105(3A):1S, 1998.

12. Mellergard M. Only extremely tired? *Ugeskrift for Laeger* 159(31):4769, 1997.

13. Sibbald B. Chronic fatigue syndrome comes out of the closet. *CMAJ* 159(5):537-541, 1998.

14. Caplan C. Chronic fatigue syndrome or just plain tired? *CMAJ* 159(5):519-520, 1998.

15. Streeten DH. The nature of chronic fatigue. *JAMA* 280(12):1094-1095, 1998.

16. Delbanco TL, Daley J, Hartman EE. A 56-year-old woman with chronic fatigue syndrome, 1 year later. *JAMA* 280(4):372, 1998.

17. Joyce J, Rabe-Hesketh S, Wessely S. Reviewing the reviews: The example of chronic fatigue syndrome. *JAMA* 280(3):264-266, 1998.

18. Nisenbaum R, Reyes M, Mawle AC, Reeves WC. Factor analysis of unexplained severe fatigue and interrelated symptoms: Overlap with criteria for chronic fatigue syndrome. *American Journal of Epidemiology* 148(1):72-77, 1998.

19. Komaroff AL, Buchwald DS. Chronic fatigue syndrome: An update. *Annual Revue of Medicine* 49:1-13, 1998.

20. Tuck I, Human N. The experience of living with chronic fatigue syndrome. *Journal of Psychosocial Nursing & Mental Health Services* 36(2):15-19, 1998.

21. Harrigan P. Controversy continues over chronic fatigue syndrome. *Lancet* 351(9102):574, 1998.

22. Hartz AJ, Kuhn EM, Levine PH. Characteristics of fatigued persons associated with features of chronic fatigue syndrome. *Journal of Chronic Fatigue Syndrome* 4(3):71-97, 1998.

23. Franklin A. How I manage chronic fatigue syndrome. *Archives of Disease in Childhood* 79(4):375-378, 1998.

24. Levine PH. What we know about chronic fatigue syndrome and its relevance to the practicing physician. *American Journal of Medicine* 105(3A):100S-103S, 1998.

25. McCluskey DR. Chronic fatigue syndrome: Its cause and a strategy for management. *Comprehensive Therapy* 24(8):357-363. 1998.

26. Kenner C. Fibromyalgia and chronic fatigue: The holistic perspective. *Holistic Nursing Practice* 12(3):55-63, 1998.

27. Fuller NS, Morrison RE. Chronic fatigue syndrome: Helping patients cope with this enigmatic illness. *Postgraduate Medicine* 103(1):175-176, 179-184, 1998.

28. Goshorn RK. Chronic fatigue syndrome: A review for clinicians. *Seminars in Neurology* 18(2):237-242, 1998.

29. Lapp CW, Hyman HL. Diagnosis of chronic fatigue syndrome. *Archives of Internal Medicine* 157(22):2663-2664, 1997.

30. Komaroff AL. A 56-year-old woman with chronic fatigue syndrome. *JAMA* 278(14):1179-1185, 1997.

31. Lipkin DM, Papernik M, Kaan R. Chronic fatigue. *American Journal of Psychiatry* 154(9):1322, 1997.

32. Miro O, Font C, Fernandez-Sola J, Casademont J, Pedrol E, Grau JM, Urbano-Marquez A. Chronic fatigue syndrome: Study of the clinical course of 28 cases. *Medicina Clinica* 108(15):561-565, 1997.

33. Bertolin JM, Calvo J. Chronic fatigue syndrome. To be or not to be? *Medicina Clinica* 108(15):577-579, 1997.

34. Houde SC, Kampfe-Leacher R. Chronic fatigue syndrome: An update for clinicians in primary care. *Nurse Practitioner* 22(7):30, 35-6, 39-40, 1997.

35. Hadler NM. Fibromyalgia, chronic fatigue, and other iatrogenic diagnostic algorithms: Do some labels escalate illness in vulnerable patients? *Postgraduate Medicine* 102(2):161-162, 165-166, 171-172, 1997.

36. Chester AC. Chronic fatigue syndrome criteria in patients with other forms of unexplained chronic fatigue. *Journal of Psychiatric Research* 31(1):45-50, 1997.

37. Salit IE. Precipitating factors for the chronic fatigue syndrome. *Journal of Psychiatric Research* 31(1):59-65, 1997.

38. Baschetti R. Etiology of chronic fatigue syndrome. *American Journal of Medicine* 102(4):422-423, 1997.

39. Cook NF, Boore JR. Managing patients suffering from acute and chronic fatigue. *British Journal of Nursing* 6(14):811-815, 1997.

40. DeLuca J, Johnson SK, Ellis SP, Natelson BH. Sudden vs. gradual onset of chronic fatigue syndrome differentiates individuals on cognitive and psychiatric measures. *Journal of Psychiatric Research* 31(1):83-90, 1997.

41. Sharpe M, Chalder T, Palmer I, Wessely S. Chronic fatigue syndrome: A practical guide to assessment and management. *General Hospital Psychiatry* 19(3):185-199, 1997.

42. Simpson M, Bennett A, Holland P. Chronic fatigue syndrome/myalgic encephalomyelitis as a twentieth-century disease: Analytic challenges. *Journal of Analytical Psychology* 42(2):191-199, 1997.

43. Heyll U, Wachauf P, Senger V, Diewitz M. Definition of "chronic fatigue syndrome" (CFS). *Medizinische Klinik* 92(4):221-227, 1997.

44. Suarez-Lozano I. Isolated general malaise of unknown origin: A new syndrome. *Anales de Medicina Interna* 14(4):209-210, 1997; Teran Diaz E. *Anales de Medicina Interna* 13(10):467-470, 1996.

45. Plioplys AV, Plioplys S, Davis JS IV. Meeting the frustrations of chronic fatigue syndrome. *Hospital Practice* 32(6):147-150, 153-156, 160-161, 1997.

46. de Loos WS. Chronic fatigue syndrome: Fatigue of unknown origin. *European Journal of Clinical Investigation* 27(4):268-269, 1997.

47. Dickinson CJ. Chronic fatigue syndrome: Aetiological aspects. *European Journal of Clinical Investigation* 27(4):257-267, 1997.

48. Salit IE. The chronic fatigue syndrome: a position paper. *The Journal of Rheumatology* 23(3):540-544, 1996.

49. Wessely S. Chronic fatigue syndrome. Summary of a report of a joint committee of the Royal College of Physicians, Psychiatrists and General Practitioners. *Journal of the Royal College of Physicians of London* 30(6):497-504, 1996.

50. Hickie I, Lloyd A, Wakefield D, Ricci C. Is there a postinfection fatigue syndrome? *Australian Family Physician* 25(12):1847-1852, 1996.

51. Lieb K, Dammann G, Berger M, Bauer J. Chronic fatigue syndrome. Definition, diagnostic measures and therapeutic possibilities. *Nervenarzt* 67(9):711-720, 1996.

52. Buchwald D, Umali J, Pearlman T, Kith P, Ashley R, Wener M. Postinfectious chronic fatigue: A distinct syndrome? *Clinical Infectious Diseases* 23(2):385-387, 1996; Chalder T, Power MJ, Wessely S. Chronic fatigue in the community: A question of attribution. *Psychological Medicine* 26(4):791-800, 1996.

53. Ross E. The history and treatment of chronic fatigue syndrome. *Nursing Times* 92(44):34-36, 1996.

54. Mulube M. Myths dispelled about chronic fatigue syndrome. *British Medical Journal* 313(7061):839, 1996.

55. Gompels MM, Spickett GP. Chronic fatigue, arthralgia, and malaise. *Annals of Rheumatological Diseases* 55(8):502-503, 1996.

56. Butler C, Rollnick S. Missing the meaning and provoking resistance; a case of myalgic encephalomyelitis. *Family Practice* 13(1):106-109, 1996.

57. van Waveren EK. The rise and fall of the chronic fatigue syndrome as defined by Holmes et al. *Medical Hypotheses* 46(2):63-66, 1996.

58. Hausotter W. Expert assessment of chronic fatigue syndrome. *Versicherungsmedizin* 48(2):57-59, 1996.

59. Hakimi R. Chronic fatigue syndrome—also an insurance medicine problem. *Versicherungsmedizin* 48(2):59-61, 1996.

60. Dyck D, Allen S, Barron J, Marchi J, Price BA, Spavor L, Tateishi S. Management of chronic fatigue syndrome: case study. *AAOHN Journal* 44(2):85-92, 1996.

61. MacDonald KL, Osterholm MT, LeDell KH, White KE, Schenck CH, Chao CC, Persing DH, Johnson RC, Barker JM, Peterson PK. A case-control study to assess possible triggers and cofactors in chronic fatigue syndrome. *American Journal of Medicine* 100(5):548-554, 1996.

62. Komaroff AL, Fagioli LR, Geiger AM, Doolittle TH, Lee J, Kornish RJ, Gleit MA, Guerriero RT. An examination of the working case definition of chronic fatigue syndrome. *American Journal of Medicine* 100(1):56-64, 1996.

Ciguatera

1. Pearn JH. Chronic ciguatera: One organic cause of the chronic fatigue syndrome. *Journal of Chronic Fatigue Syndrome* 2(2/3):29-34, 1996.

2. Pearn JH. Chronic fatigue syndrome: Chronic ciguatera poisoning as a differential diagnosis. *Medical Journal of Australia* 166(6):309-310, 1997.

Circadian rhythms

1. van de Luit L, van der Meulen J, Cleophas TJ, Zwinderman AH. Amplified amplitudes of circadian rhythms and nighttime hypotension in patients with chronic fatigue syndrome: Improvement by inomapil but not by melatonin. *Angiology* 49(11):903-908, 1998.

2. Williams G, Pirmohamed J, Minors D, Waterhouse J, Buchan I, Arendt J. Dissociation of body temperature and melatonin secretion circadian rhythms in patients with chronic fatigue syndrome. *Clinical Physiology* 16(4):327-337, 1996.

3. Hamilos DL, Nutter D, Gershtenson J, Redmond DP, Clementi JD, Schmaling KB, Make BJ, Jones JF. Core body temperature is normal in chronic fatigue syndrome. *Biological Psychiatry* 43(4):293-302, 1998.

Circulating immune complexes

1. Bates DW, Buchwald D, Lee J, Kith P, Doolittle T, Rutherford C, Churchill WH, Schur PH, Werner M, Wybenga D et al. Clinical laboratory test findings in patients with chronic fatigue syndrome. *Archives of Internal Medicine* 155:97-103, 1995.

2. Behan PO, Behan WHM, Bell EJ. The postviral fatigue syndrome—An analysis of the findings in 50 cases. *Journal of Infection* 10:211-22, 1985.

3. Borysiewicz LK, Haworth SJ, Cohen J et al. Epstein-Barr virus—specific immune defects in patients with persistent symptoms following infectious mononucleosis. *Quarterly Journal of Medicine* 58:111-121, 1986.

4. Straus SE, Tosato G, Armstrong G et al. Persisting illness and fatigue in adults with evidence of Epstein-Barr virus infection. *Annals of Internal Medicine* 102:7-16, 1985.

5. Natelson BH, LaManca JJ, Denny TN, Vladutiu A, Oleske J, Hill N, Bergen MT, Korn L, Hay J. Immunologic parameters in chronic fatigue syndrome, major depression, and multiple sclerosis. *American Journal of Medicine* 105(3A): 43S-49S, 1998.

6. Mawle AC, Nisenbaum R, Dobbins JG, Gary HE Jr, Stewart JA, Reyes M, Steele L, Schmid DS, Reeves WC. Immune responses associated with chronic fatigue syndrome: A case-control study. *The Journal of Infectious Diseases* 175(1):136-141, 1997.

7. Buchwald D, Wener MH, Pearlman T, Kith P. Markers of inflammation and immune activation in chronic fatigue and chronic fatigue syndrome. *The Journal of Rheumatology* 24(2):372-376, 1997.

Cognitive behavioral therapy

1. Demitrack MA. Chronic fatigue syndrome and fibromyalgia. Dilemmas in diagnosis and clinical management. *Psychiatric Clinics of North America* 21(3): 671-692, 1998.

2. Sharpe M. Cognitive behavior therapy for chronic fatigue syndrome: Efficacy and implications. *American Journal of Medicine* 105(3A):104S-109S, 1998.

3. Sharpe M. Cognitive behavior therapy for chronic fatigue syndrome. *American Journal of Psychiatry* 155(10):1461-1462, 1998.

4. Sharpe M. Cognitive behavior therapy for functional somatic complaints. The example of chronic fatigue syndrome. *Psychosomatics* 38(4):356-362, 1997.

5. Wilhelmsen I, Bodtker J. Chronic fatigue syndrome and cognitive therapy. *Tidsskrift for Den Norske Laegeforening* 116(13):1615, 1996.

6. Ho-Yen DO. Cognitive behavior therapy for the chronic fatigue syndrome. Patients' beliefs about their illness were probably not a major factor. *British Medical Journal* 312(7038):1097-1098, 1996.

7. Eaton KK. Cognitive behaviour therapy for the chronic fatigue syndrome. Use an interdisciplinary approach. *British Medical Journal* 312(7038):1097; discussion 1098, 1996.

8. Lawrie SM. Cognitive behaviour therapy for the chronic fatigue syndrome. Essential elements of the treatment must be identified. *British Medical Journal* 312(7038):1097; discussion 1098, 1996.

9. Chilton SA. Cognitive behaviour therapy for the chronic fatigue syndrome. Evening primrose oil and magnesium have been shown to be effective. *British Medical Journal* 312(7038):1096; discussion 1098, 1996.

10. Hamre HJ. Chronic fatigue syndrome and cognitive therapy. *Tidsskrift for Den Norske Laegeforening* 116(12):1503, 1996.

11. Marlin RG, Anchel H, Gibson JC, Goldberg WM, Swinton M. An evaluation of multidisciplinary intervention for chronic fatigue syndrome with long-term follow-up, and a comparison with unrelated controls. *American Journal of Medicine* 105(3A):110S-114S, 1998.

12. Deale A, Chalder T, Marks I, Wessely S. Cognitive behavior therapy for chronic fatigue syndrome: A randomized controlled trial. *American Journal of Psychiatry* 154(3):408-414, 1997.

13. Sharpe M, Hawton K, Simkin S, Surawy C, Hackmann A, Klimes I, Peto T, Warrell D, Seagroatt V. Cognitive behaviour therapy for the chronic fatigue syndrome: A randomized controlled trial. *British Medical Journal* 312(7022):22-26, 1996.

Connective tissue and rheumatologic disorders

1. Fiore G, Giacovazzo F, Giacovazzo M. Three cases of dermatomyositis erroneously diagnosed as "chronic fatigue syndrome." *European Review of Medicine & Pharmacological Sciences* 1(6):193-195, 1997.

2. Nishikai M, Akiya K, Tojo T, Onoda N, Tani M, Shimizu K. "Seronegative" Sjögren's syndrome manifested as a subset of chronic fatigue syndrome. *British Journal of Rheumatology* 35(5):471-474, 1996.

3. Barendregt PJ, Visser MR, Smets EM, Tulen JH, van den Meiracker AH, Boomsma F, Markusse HM. Fatigue in primary Sjögren's syndrome. *Annals of Rheumatic Diseases* 57(5):291-295, 1998.

4. Asim M, Turney JH. The female patient with faints and fatigue: Don't forget Sjögren's syndrome. *Nephrology, Dialysis, Transplantation* 12(7):1516-1517, 1997.

5. Wang B, Gladman DD, Urowitz MB. Fatigue in lupus is not correlated with disease activity. *The Journal of Rheumatology* 25(5):892-895, 1998.

6. Jones SD, Koh WH, Steiner A, Garrett SL, Calin A. Fatigue in ankylosing spondylitis: Its prevalence and relationship to disease activity, sleep, and other factors. *The Journal of Rheumatology* 23(3):487-490, 1996.

7. Wolfe F, Hawley DJ, Wilson K. The prevalence and meaning of fatigue in rheumatic disease. *The Journal of Rheumatology* 23(8):1407-1417, 1996.

8. Huyser BA, Parker JC, Thoreson R, Smarr KL, Johnson JC, Hoffman R. Predictors of subjective fatigue among individuals with rheumatoid arthritis. *Arthritis & Rheumatism* 41(12):2230-2237, 1998.

9. Riemsma RP, Rasker JJ, Taal E, Griep EN, Wouters JM, Wiegman O. Fatigue in rheumatoid arthritis: The role of self-efficacy and problematic social support. *British Journal of Rheumatology* 37(10):1042-1046, 1998.

10. Stone AA, Broderick JE, Porter LS, Kaell AT. The experience of rheumatoid arthritis pain and fatigue: Examining momentary reports and correlates over one week. *Arthritis Care & Research* 10(3):185-193, 1997.

Coronary artery disease

1. Vilikus Z, Mareckova H, Janatkova I, Krystufkova O, Barackova M, Boudova L, Brandejsky P, Fucikova T. Risk factors for ischemic heart disease in patients with chronic fatigue syndrome. *Sbornik Lekarsky* 99(1):53-61, 1998.

2. McGovern PG, Shahar E, Folsom AR, Rosamond WD. No relation between excess fatigue and asymptomatic carotid atherosclerosis. *Epidemiology* 7(6):638-40, 1996.

Cytokines

1. Patarca R, Sandler D, Walling J, Klimas NG, Fletcher MA. Assessment of immune mediator expression levels in biological fluids and cells: a critical appraisal. *Critical Reviews in Oncogenesis* 6(2):117-149, 1995.

2. Vollmer-Conna U, Lloyd A, Hickie I, Wakefield D. Chronic fatigue syndrome: An immunological perspective. *Australian & New Zealand Journal of Psychiatry* 32(4):523-527, 1998.

3. Sheng WS, Hu S, Lamkin A, Peterson PK, Chao CC. Susceptibility to immunologically mediated fatigue in C57BL/6 versus Balb/c mice. *Clinical Immunology & Immunopathology* 81(2):161-167, 1996.

4. Rook GA, Zumla A. Gulf War syndrome: Is it due to a systemic shift in cytokine balance towards a Th2 profile? *Lancet* 349(9068):1831-1833, 1997.

5. Andersson M, Bagby JR, Dyrehag L-E, Gottfries C-G. Effects of staphylococcus toxoid vaccine in patients with fibromyalgia/chronic fatigue syndrome. *European Journal of Pain* 2:133-142, 1998.

Demographics

1. Fitzgibbon EJ, Murphy D, O'Shea K, Kelleher C. Chronic debilitating fatigue in Irish general practice: A survey of general practitioners' experience. *British Journal of General Practice* 47(423):618-622, 1997.

2. Versluis RG, de Waal MW, Opmeer C, Petri H, Springer MP. Prevalence of chronic fatigue syndrome in 4 family practices in Leiden. *Nederlands Tijdschrift voor Geneeskunde* 141(31):1523-1526, 1997.

3. Van Mens-Verhulst J, Bensing J. Distinguishing between chronic and non-chronic fatigue, the role of gender and age. *Social Science & Medicine* 47(5): 621-634, 1998.

4. Van Mens-Verhulst J, Bensing JM. Sex differences in persistent fatigue. *Women & Health* 26(3):51-70, 1997.

5. Versluis RG, de Waal MW, Opmeer C, Petri H, Springer MP. Prevalence of chronic fatigue syndrome in 4 family practices in Leiden. *Nederlands Tijdschrift voor Geneeskunde* 141(31):1523-1526, 1997.

6. Levine PH, Snow PG, Ranum BA, Paul C, Holmes MJ. Epidemic neuromysthenia and chronic fatigue syndrome in West Otago, New Zealand. A 10-year follow-up. *Archives of Internal Medicine* 157(7):750-754, 1997.

7. Euga R, Chalder T, Deale A, Wessely S. A comparison of the characteristics of chronic fatigue syndrome in primary and tertiary care. *British Journal of Psychiatry* 168(1):121-126, 1996.

8. Loge JH, Ekeberg O, Kaasa S. Fatigue in the general Norwegian population: Normative data and associations. *Journal of Psychosomatic Research* 45:53-65, 1998.

9. Steele L, Dobbins JG, Fukuda K, Reyes M, Randall B, Koppelman M, Reeves WC. The epidemiology of chronic fatigue in San Francisco. *American Journal of Medicine* 105(3A):83S-90S, 1998.

Dental amalgam fillings

1. Malt UF, Nerdrum P, Oppedal B, Gundersen R, Holte M, Lone J. Physical and mental problems attributed to dental amalgam fillings: A descriptive study of 99 self-referred patients compared with 272 controls. *Psychosomatic Medicine* 59(1):32-41, 1997.
2. Langworth S, Stromberg R. A case of high mercury exposure from dental amalgam. *European Journal of Oral Science* 104(3):320-321, 1996.

Disability

1. Bombardier CH, Buchwald D. Chronic fatigue, chronic fatigue syndrome, and fibromyalgia. Disability and health-care use. *Medical Care* 34(9):924-930, 1996.
2. Versluis RG, de Waal MW, Opmeer C, Petri H, Springer MP. Prevalence of chronic fatigue syndrome in four family practices in Leiden. *Nederlands Tijdschrift voor Geneeskunde* 141(31):1523-1526, 1997.
3. Buchwald D, Pearlman T, Umali J, Schmaling K, Katon W. Functional status in patients with chronic fatigue syndrome, other fatiguing illnesses, and healthy individuals. *American Journal of Medicine* 101(4):364-370, 1996.
4. Komaroff AL, Fagioli LR, Doolittle TH, Gandek B, Gleit MA, Guerriero RT, Kornish RJ II, Ware NC, Ware JE Jr, Bates DW. Health status in patients with chronic fatigue syndrome and in general population and disease comparison groups. *American Journal of Medicine* 101(3):281-290, 1996.
5. Christodoulou C, DeLuca J, Lange G, Johnson SK, Sisto SA, Korn L, Natelson BH. Relation between neuropsychological impairment and functional disability in patients with chronic fatigue syndrome. *Journal of Neurology, Neurosurgery & Psychiatry* 64(4):431-434, 1998.

Energy Expenditure

1. Watson, WS, McMillan DC, Chaudhuri A, Behan PO. Increased resting energy expenditure in the chronic fatigue syndrome. *Journal of Chronic Fatigue Syndrome* 4(4):3-14, 1998.

Enteroviruses

1. Fohlman J, Friman G, Tuvemo T. Enterovirus infections in new disguise. *Lakartidningen* 94(28-29):2555-2560, 1997.
2. Galbraith DN, Nairn C, Clements GB. Evidence for enteroviral persistence in humans. *Journal of General Virology* 78 (Pt 2):307-312, 1997.
3. Hill WM. Are echoviruses still orphan? *British Journal of Biomedical Science* 53(3):221-226, 1996.

4. Buchwald D, Ashley RL, Pearlman T, Kith P, Komaroff AL. Viral serologies in patients with chronic fatigue and chronic fatigue syndrome. *Journal of Medical Virology* 50(1):25-30, 1996.

5. Lindh G, Samuelson A, Hedlund KO, Evengard B, Lindquist L, Ehrnst A. No findings of enteroviruses in Swedish patients with chronic fatigue syndrome. *Scandinavian Journal of Infectious Diseases* 28(3):305-307, 1996.

6. McArdle A, McArdle F, Jackson MJ, Page SF, Fahal I, Edwards RH. Investigation by polymerase chain reaction of enteroviral infection in patients with chronic fatigue syndrome. *Clinical Science* 90(4):295-300, 1996.

Epidemiology

1. Sutton GC. "Too tired to go to the support group": A health needs assessment of myalgic encephalomyelitis. *Journal of Public Health Medicine* 18(3): 343-349, 1996.

2. Fukuda K, Dobbins JG, Wilson LJ, Dunn RA, Wilcox K, Smallwood D. An epidemiologic study of fatigue with relevance for the chronic fatigue syndrome. *Journal of Psychiatric Research* 31(1):19-29, 1997.

3. Fitzgibbon EJ, Murphy D, O'Shea K, Kelleher C. Chronic debilitating fatigue in Irish general practice: A survey of general practitioners' experience. *British Journal of General Practice* 47(423):618-622, 1997.

4. Wessely S, Chalder T, Hirsch S, Wallace P, Wright D. The prevalence and morbidity of chronic fatigue and chronic fatigue syndrome: A prospective primary care study. *American Journal of Public Health* 87(9):1449-1455, 1997.

5. Versluis RG, de Waal MW, Opmeer C, Petri H, Springer MP. Prevalence of chronic fatigue syndrome in four family practices in Leiden. *Nederlands Tijdschrift voor Geneeskunde* 141(31):1523-1526, 1997.

6. Bazelmans E, Vercoulen JH, Galama JM, van Weel C, van der Meer JW, Bleijenberg G. Prevalence of chronic fatigue syndrome and primary fibromyalgia syndrome in the Netherlands. *Nederlands Tijdschrift voor Geneeskunde* 141(31): 1520-1523, 1997.

7. de Jong LW, Prins JB, Fiselier TJ, Weemaes CM, Meijer-van den Bergh EM, Bleijenberg G. Chronic fatigue syndrome in young persons. *Nederlands Tijdschrift voor Geneeskunde* 141(31):1513-1516, 1997.

8. Minowa M, Jiamo M. Descriptive epidemiology of chronic fatigue syndrome based on a nationwide survey in Japan. *American Journal of Epidemiology* 6(2):75-80, 1996.

9. Levine PH, Snow PG, Ranum BA, Paul C, Holmes MJ. Epidemic neuromyasthenia and chronic fatigue syndrome in West Otago, New Zealand. A 10-year follow-up. *Archives of Internal Medicine* 157(7):750-754, 1997.

10. Levine PH. Epidemiologic advances in chronic fatigue syndrome. *Journal of Psychiatric Research* 31(1):7-18, 1997.

11. White PD, Thomas JM, Amess J, Crawford DH, Grover SA, Kangro HO, Clare AW. Incidence, risk and prognosis of acute and chronic fatigue syndromes and psychiatric disorders after glandular fever. *British Journal of Psychiatry* 173:475-481, 1998.

12. Jason LA, Wagner L, Rosenthal S, Goodlatte J, Lipkin D, Papernik M, Plioplys S, Plioplys V. Estimating the prevalence of chronic fatigue syndrome among nurses. *American Journal of Medicine* 105(3A):91S-93S, 1998.

Exercise

1. Blackwood SK, MacHale SM, Power MJ, Goodwin GM, Lawrie SM. Effects of exercise on cognitive and motor function in chronic fatigue syndrome and depression. *Journal of Neurology, Neurosurgery & Psychiatry* 65(4):541-546, 1998.

2. LaManca JJ, Sisto SA, DeLuca J, Johnson SK, Lange G, Pareja J, Cook S, Natelson BH. Influence of exhaustive treadmill exercise on cognitive functioning in chronic fatigue syndrome. *American Journal of Medicine* 105(3A):59S-65S, 1998.

3. Rowbottom DG, Keast D, Green S, Kakulas B, Morton AR. The case history of an elite ultra-endurance cyclist who developed chronic fatigue syndrome. *Medicine & Science in Sports & Exercise* 30(9):1345-1348, 1998.

4. Samii A, Wassermann EM, Ikoma K, Mercuri B, George MS, O'Fallon A, Dale JK, Straus SE, Hallett M. Decreased postexercise facilitation of motor evoked potentials in patients with chronic fatigue syndrome or depression. *Neurology* 47(6):1410-1414, 1996.

5. McCully KK, Sisto SA, Natelson BH. Use of exercise for treatment of chronic fatigue syndrome. *American Journal of Sports Medicine* 21(1):35-48, 1996.

6. Sisto SA, Tapp WN, LaManca JJ, Ling W, Korn LR, Nelson AJ, Natelson BH. Physical activity before and after exercise in women with chronic fatigue syndrome. *Quarterly Journal of Medicine* 91(7):465-473, 1998.

7. Sisto SA, LaManca JJ, Cordero DL, Bergen MT, Ellis SP, Drastal S, Boda WL, Tapp WN, Natelson BH. Metabolic and cardiovascular effects of a progressive exercise test in patients with chronic fatigue syndrome. *American Journal of Medicine* 100(6):634-640, 1996.

8. Mock V, Ropka ME, Rhodes VA, Pickett M, Grimm PM, McDaniel R, Lin EM, Allocca P, Dienemann JA, Haisfield-Wolfe ME, Stewart KJ, McCorkle R. Establishing mechanisms to conduct multi-institutional research—Fatigue in patients with cancer: An exercise intervention. *Oncology Nursing Forum* 25(8):1391-1397, 1998.

9. Fulcher KY, White PD. Randomised controlled trial of graded exercise in patients with the chronic fatigue syndrome. *British Medical Journal* 314(7095): 1647-1652, 1997.

10. Goudsmit E. Treating chronic fatigue with exercise. Exercise, and rest, should be tailored to individual needs. *British Medical Journal* 317(7158):599-600, 1998.

11. Michael A. Treating chronic fatigue with exercise. Exercise improves mood and sleep. *British Medical Journal* 317(7158):600, 1998.

12. Baschetti R. Treating chronic fatigue with exercise. Results are contradictory for patients meeting different diagnostic criteria. *British Medical Journal* 317(7158):600, 1998.

13. Goudsmit EM. Graded exercise in chronic fatigue syndrome. Chronic fatigue syndrome is a heterogeneous condition. *British Medical Journal* 315(7113): 948, 1997.

14. Sadler M. Graded exercise in chronic fatigue syndrome. Patients were a selected group. *British Medical Journal* 315(7113):947-948, 1997.

15. Franklin AJ. Graded exercise in chronic fatigue syndrome. Including patients who rated themselves as a little better would have altered results. *British Medical Journal* 315(7113):947-948, 1997.

16. Shepherd C, Macintyre A. Graded exercise in chronic fatigue syndrome. Patients should have an initial period of rest before gradual increase in activity. *British Medical Journal* 315(7113):947-948, 1997.

17. Lapp CW. Exercise limits in chronic fatigue syndrome. *American Journal of Medicine* 103(1):83-84, 1997.

18. Elliot DL, Goldberg L, Loveless MO. Graded exercise testing and chronic fatigue syndrome. *American Journal of Medicine* 103(1):84-86, 1997.

Familial chronic fatigue syndrome

1. Levine PH, Whiteside TL, Friberg D, Bryant J, Colclough G, Herberman RB. Dysfunction of natural killer activity in a family with chronic fatigue syndrome. *Clinical Immunology & Immunopathology* 88(1):96-104, 1998.

2. George DK, Evans RM, Gunn IR. Familial chronic fatigue. *Postgraduate Medical Journal* 73(859):311-313, 1997.

Fatigue

1. Ream E, Richardson A. Fatigue: A concept analysis. *International Journal of Nursing Studies* 33(5):519-529, 1996.

2. Tiesinga LJ, Dassen TW, Halfens RJ. Fatigue: A summary of the definitions, dimensions, and indicators. *Nursing Diagnosis* 7(2):51-62, 1996.

3. Groopman JE. Fatigue in cancer and HIV/AIDS. *Oncology* 12(3):335-344, 1998.

4. White PD. The relationship between infection and fatigue. *Journal of Psychosomatic Research* 43(4):345-350, 1997.

5. Llewelyn MB. Assessing the fatigued patient. *British Journal of Hospital Medicine* 55(3):125-129, 1996.

6. Shapiro CM. Fatigue: How many types and how common? *Journal of Psychosomatic Research* 45:1-3, 1998.

Fibromyalgia

1. Bennett R. Fibromyalgia, chronic fatigue syndrome, and myofascial pain. *Current Opinions in Rheumatology* 10(2):95-103, 1998.

2. Slavkin HC. Chronic disabling diseases and disorders: The challenges of fibromyalgia. *Journal of the American Dental Association* 128(11):1583-1589, 1997.

3. Celiker R, Borman P, Oktem F, Gokce-Kutsal Y, Basgoze O. Psychological disturbance in fibromyalgia: Relation to pain severity. *Clinical Rheumatology* 16(2):179-184, 1997.

4. Hadler NM. Is fibromyalgia a useful diagnostic label? *Cleveland Clinical Journal of Medicine* 63(2):85-87, 1996.

5. MacFarlane GJ, Croft PR, Schollum J, Silman AJ. Widespread pain: Is an improved classification possible? *The Journal of Rheumatology* 23(9):1628-1632, 1996.

6. Kennedy M, Felson DT. A prospective long-term study of fibromyalgia syndrome. *Arthritis & Rheumatism* 39(4):682-685, 1996.

7. Park JH, Phothimat P, Oates CT, Hernanz-Schulman M, Olsen NJ. Use of P-31 magnetic resonance spectroscopy to detect metabolic abnormalities in muscles of patients with fibromyalgia. *Arthritis & Rheumatism* 41(3):406-413, 1998.

8. Bazelmans E, Vercoulen JH, Galama JM, van Weel C, van der Meer JW, Bleijenberg G. Prevalence of chronic fatigue syndrome and primary fibromyalgia syndrome in the Netherlands. *Nederlands Tijdschrift voor Geneeskunde* 141(31): 1520-1523, 1997.

9. Chambers CR. Fireworks over fibromyalgia, CFS, and IBS. *Postgraduate Medicine* 102(6):43, 1997; Pocinki AG. *Postgraduate Medicine* 102(6):43, 1997; Sabal N. *Postgraduate Medicine* 102(6):44, 1997; Vree R. *Postgraduate Medicine* 102(6):44, 1997.

10. Kelly MC. Fibromyalgia syndrome. *Irish Medical Journal* 90(1):14-16, 1997.

11. Goldenberg DL. Fibromyalgia, chronic fatigue syndrome, and myofascial pain syndrome. *Current Opinions in Rheumatology* 9(2):135-143, 1997.

12. Wallace DJ. The fibromyalgia syndrome. *Annals of Medicine* 29(1):9-21, 1997.

13. Buchwald D. Fibromyalgia and chronic fatigue syndrome: Similarities and differences. *Rheumatic Disease Clinics of North America* 22(2):219-243, 1996.

14. Hoffmann A, Linder R, Kroger B, Schnabel A, Kruger GR. Fibromyalgia syndrome and chronic fatigue syndrome. Similarities and differences. *Deutsche Medizinische Wochenschrift* 121(38):1165-1168, 1996.

15. Hadler NM. If you have to prove you are ill, you can't get well. The object lesson of fibromyalgia. *Spine* 21(20):2397-2400, 1996.

16. Ben-Zion I, Shieber A, Buskila D. Psychiatric aspects of fibromyalgia syndrome. *Harefuah* 131(3-4):127-129, 1996.

17. Affleck G, Tennen H, Urrows S, Higgins P, Abeles M, Hall C, Karoly P, Newton C. Fibromyalgia and women's pursuit of personal goals: A daily process analysis. *Health Psychology* 17(1):40-47, 1998.

18. Schaefer KM. Health patients of women with fibromyalgia. *Journal of Advanced Nursing* 26(3):565-571, 1997.

19. Reid GJ, Lang BA, McGrath PJ. Primary juvenile fibromyalgia: Psychological adjustment, family functioning, coping, and functional disability. *Arthritis & Rheumatism* 40(4):752-760, 1997.

20. Kurtze N, Gundersen KT, Svebak S. The role of anxiety and depression in fatigue and patterns of pain among subgroups of fibromyalgia patients. *British Journal of Medicine and Psychology* 71(Pt 2):185-194, 1998.

21. Scharf MB, Hauck M, Stover R, McDannold M, Berkowitz D. Effect of gamma-hydroxybutyrate on pain, fatigue, and the alpha sleep anomaly in patients with fibromyalgia. Preliminary report. *The Journal of Rheumatology* 25(10):1986-1990, 1998.

22. Moldofsky H, Lue FA, Mously C, Roth-Schechter B, Reynolds WJ. The effect of zolpidem in patients with fibromyalgia: A dose ranging, double-blind, placebo-controlled, modified crossover study. *The Journal of Rheumatology* 23(3): 529-533, 1996.

Gastrointestinal pathology

1. Korszun A, Papadopoulos E, Demitrack M, Engleberg C, Crofford L. The relationship between temporomandibular disorders and stress-associated syndromes. *Oral Surgery, Oral Medicine, Oral Pathology, Oral Radiology, & Endodontics* 86(4):416-420, 1998.

2. Gomborone JE, Gorard DA, Dewsnap PA, Libby GW, Farthing MJ. Prevalence of irritable bowel syndrome in chronic fatigue. *Journal of the Royal College of Physicians of London* 30(6):512-513, 1996.

3. Chambers CR. *Postgraduate Medicine* 102(6):43, 1997; Pocinki AG. Fireworks over fibromyalgia, CFS, and IBS. *Postgraduate Medicine* 102(6):43, 1997; Sabal N. *Postgraduate Medicine* 102(6):44, 1997; Vree R. *Postgraduate Medicine* 102(6):44, 1997.

4. Hyman H, Wasser TE. Gastrointestinal manifestations of chronic fatigue syndrome (CFS): Symptom perceptions and quality of life. *Journal of Chronic Fatigue Syndrome* 4(1):43-52, 1998.

5. Empson M. Celiac disease or chronic fatigue syndrome—Can the current CDC working case definition discriminate? *American Journal of Medicine* 105(1): 79-80, 1998.

6. Corrado G, Riezzo G, Rea P, Pacchiarotti C, Cavaliere M, Cardi E. Normal gastric emptying and myoelectrical activity in an adolescent with chronic fatigue syndrome. *Italian Journal of Gastroenterology & Hepatology* 30(4):444-445, 1998.

Glandular fever

1. White PD, Thomas JM, Amess J, Crawford DH, Grover SA, Kangro HO, Clare AW. Incidence, risk and prognosis of acute and chronic fatigue syndromes and psychiatric disorders after glandular fever. *British Journal of Psychiatry* 173:475-481, 1998.

2. White PD, Dash AR, Thomas JM. Poor concentration and the ability to process information after glandular fever. *Journal of Psychosomatic Research* 44(2):269-278, 1998.

Gulf War syndrome

1. The Iowa Persian Gulf Study Group. Self-reported illness and health status among Gulf War veterans. A population-based study. *JAMA* 277(3):238-245, 1997.
2. Fiedler N, Kipen H, Natelson B, Ottenweller J. Chemical sensitivities and the Gulf War: Department of Veterans Affairs research center in basic and clinical studies of environmental hazards. *Regulatory Toxicology & Pharmacology* 24(1 Pt 2):S129-S138, 1996.
3. Hyams KC. Lessons derived from evaluating Gulf War syndrome: Suggested guidelines for investigating outbreaks of new diseases. *Psychosomatic Medicine* 60(2):137-139, 1998.
4. Selner JC. Chamber challenges: The necessity of objective observation. *Regulatory Toxicology & Pharmacology* 24(1 Pt 2):S87-S95, 1996.
5. Nicolson GL, Bruton DM Jr, Nicolson NL. Chronic fatigue illness and Operation Desert Storm. *Journal of Occupational & Environmental Medicine* 38(1):14-16, 1996.
6. Coker WJ. A review of Gulf War illness. *Journal of the Royal Naval Medical Service* 82(2):141-146, 1996.
7. Rook GA, Zumla A. Gulf War syndrome: Is it due to a systemic shift in cytokine balance towards a Th2 profile? *Lancet* 349(9068):1831-1833, 1997.
8. Malone JD, Paige-Dobson B, Ohl C, DiGiovanni C, Cunnion S, Roy MJ. Possibilities for unexplained chronic illnesses among reserve units deployed in Operation Desert Shield/Desert Storm. *Southern Medical Journal* 89(12):1147-1155, 1996.

Gynecology

1. Harlow BL, Signorello LB, Hall JE, Dailey C, Komaroff AL. Reproductive correlates of chronic fatigue syndrome. *American Journal of Medicine* 105(3A): 94S-99S, 1998.

Herpesviruses

1. Glaser R, Kiecolt-Glaser JK. Stress-associated immune modulation: Relevance to viral infections and chronic fatigue syndrome. *American Journal of Medicine* 105(3A):35S-42S, 1998.
2. Bennett BK, Hickie IB, Vollmer-Conna US, Quigley B, Brennan CM, Wakefield D, Douglas MP, Hansen GR, Tahmindjis AJ, Lloyd AR. The relationship between fatigue, psychological and immunological variables in acute infectious illness. *Australian & New Zealand Journal of Psychiatry* 32(2):180-186, 1998.
3. White PD, Thomas JM, Amess J, Crawford DH, Grover SA, Kangro HO, Clare AW. Incidence, risk and prognosis of acute and chronic fatigue syndromes and psychiatric disorders after glandular fever. *British Journal of Psychiatry* 173:475-481, 1998.
4. Schmaling KB, Jones JF. MMPI profiles of patients with chronic fatigue syndrome. *Journal of Psychosomatic Research* 40(1):67-74, 1996.

5. Buchwald D, Ashley RL, Pearlman T, Kith P, Komaroff AL. Viral serologies in patients with chronic fatigue and chronic fatigue syndrome. *Journal of Medical Virology* 50(1):25-30, 1996.

6. Martin WJ. Cellular sequences in stealth viruses. *Pathobiology* 66(2):53-58, 1998.

7. Martin WJ. Detection of RNA sequences in cultures of a stealth virus isolated from the cerebrospinal fluid of a health care worker with chronic fatigue syndrome. Case report. *Pathobiology* 65(1):57-60, 1997.

8. Martin WJ. Severe stealth virus encephalopathy following chronic-fatigue-syndrome-like illness: Clinical and histopathological features. *Pathobiology* 64(1): 1-8, 1996.

9. Martin WJ. Genetic instability and fragmentation of a stealth viral genome. *Pathobiology* 64(1):9-17, 1996.

10. Tripathy BK, Agarwal AK, Sangla KS, Singh CP, Chandra S. Infectious agents and immunological disturbances in relation to chronic fatigue syndrome. *Journal of the Association of Physicians of India* 44(5):335-338, 1996.

11. Braun DK, Dominguez G, Pellett PE. Human herpesvirus 6. *Clinical Microbiology Reviews* 10(3):521-67, 1997.

12. Marsh S, Kaplan M, Asano Y, Hoekzema D, Komaroff AL, Whitman JE Jr, Ablashi DV. Development and application of HHV-6 antigen capture assay for the detection of HHV-6 infections. *Journal of Virological Methods* 61(1-2):103-112, 1996.

13. Cuende JI, Civeira P, Diez N, Prieto J. High prevalence without reactivation of herpesvirus 6 in subjects with chronic fatigue syndrome. *Anales de Medicina Interna* 14(9):441-444, 1997.

14. Ablashi DV, Handy M, Bernbaum J, Chatlynne LG, Lapps W, Kramarsky B, Berneman ZN, Komaroff AL, Whitman JE. Propagation and characterization of human herpesvirus-7 (HHV-7) isolates in a continuous T-lymphoblastoid cell line (SUPT1). *Journal of Virological Methods* 73(2):123-140, 1998.

15. Levine PH. The use of transfer factors in chronic fatigue syndrome: Prospects and problems. *Biotherapy* 9(1-3):77-79, 1996.

16. Ablashi DV, Levine PH, De Vinci C, Whitman JE Jr, Pizza G, Viza D. The use of anti HHV-6 transfer factor for the treatment of two patients with chronic fatigue syndrome (CFS). Two case reports. *Biotherapy* 9(1-3):81-86, 1996.

17. De Vinci C, Levine PH, Pizza G, Fudenberg HH, Orens P, Pearson G, Viza D. Lessons from a pilot study of transfer factor in chronic fatigue syndrome. *Biotherapy* 9(1-3):87-90, 1996.

18. Hana I, Vrubel J, Pekarek J, Cech K. The influence of age on transfer factor treatment of cellular immunodeficiency, chronic fatigue syndrome and/or chronic viral infections. *Biotherapy* 9(1-3):91-95, 1996.

Homocysteine

1. Regland B, Andersson M, Abrahamsson L, Bagby J, Dyrehag LE, Gottfries CG. Increased concentrations of homocysteine in the cerebrospinal fluid in patients

with fibromyalgia and chronic fatigue syndrome. *Scandinavian Journal of Rheumatology* 26(4):301-307, 1997.

Hypothyroidism

1. Borysiewicz LK, Haworth SJ, Cohen J et al. Epstein-Barr virus-specific immune defects in patients with persistent symptoms following infectious mononucleosis. *Quarterly Journal of Medicine* 58:111-121, 1986.
2. Buchwald D, Komaroff AL. Review of laboratory findings for patients with chronic fatigue syndrome. *Reviews of Infectious Diseases* 13(1):S12-18, 1991.
3. Kaslow JE, Ruckner L, Onishi R. Liver extract-folic acid-cyanocobalamin vs. placebo for chronic fatigue syndrome. *Archives of Internal Medicine* 149:2501-2503, 1989.
4. Kroenke K, Wood DR, Mangelsdroff AD et al. Chronic fatigue in primary care: Prevalence, patient characteristics, and outcome. *JAMA* 260:929-934, 1988.
5. Lane TJ, Manu P, Matthews DA. Prospective diagnostic evaluation of adults with chronic fatigue. *Clinical Research* 36:714A, 1988.
6. Prieto J, Subira ML, Castilla A et al. Naloxone-reversible monocyte dysfunction in patients with chronic fatigue syndrome. *Scandinavian Journal of Immunology* 30:13-20, 1989.
7. Behan PO, Behan WHM, Bell EJ. The postviral fatigue syndrome—An analysis of the findings in 50 cases. *Journal of Infection* 10:211-222, 1985.
8. Tobi M, Morag A, Ravid Z et al. Prolonged atypical illness associated with serological evidence of persistent Epstein-Barr infection. *Lancet* 1:61-64, 1982.
9. Weinstein L. Thyroiditis and "chronic infectious mononucleosis." *New England Journal of Medicine* 317:1225-1226, 1987.
10. Dinarello CA. Biology of interleukin-1. *FASEB* 2:108-115, 1988.
11. Jones TH, Wadler S, Hupart KH. Endocrine-mediated mechanisms of fatigue during treatment with interferon-alpha. *Seminars in Oncology* 25(1 Suppl 1): 54-63, 1998.

Iceland disease

1. Lindal E, Bergmann S, Thorlacius S, Stefansson JG. Anxiety disorders: A result of long-term chronic fatigue—The psychiatric characteristics of the sufferers of Iceland disease. *Acta Neurologica Scandinavica* 96(3):158-162, 1997.

Illness beliefs

1. Lloyd AR. Chronic fatigue and chronic fatigue syndrome: Shifting boundaries and attributions. *American Journal of Medicine* 105(3A):7S-10S, 1998.
2. Fry AM, Martin M. Fatigue in the chronic fatigue syndrome: A cognitive phenomenon? *Journal of Psychosomatic Research* 41(5):415-426, 1996.
3. Bleijenberg G. Attributions and chronic fatigue. *Nederlands Tijdschrift voor Geneeskunde* 141(31):1510-1512, 1997.

4. Deale A, Chalder T, Wessely S. Illness beliefs and treatment outcome in chronic fatigue syndrome. *Journal of Psychosomatic Research* 45:77-83, 1998.

5. Ray C, Jefferies S, Weir WR. Coping and other predictors of outcome in chronic fatigue syndrome: A 1-year follow-up. *Journal of Psychosomatic Research* 43(4):405-415, 1997.

6. Heijmans MJ. Coping and adaptive outcome in chronic fatigue syndrome: Importance of illness cognitions. *Journal of Psychosomatic Research* 45:39-51, 1998.

7. Stewart D, Abbey S, Meana M, Boydell JM. What makes women tired? A community sample. *Journal of Women's Health* 7(1):69-76, 1998.

8. Hall GH, Hamilton WT, Round AP. Increased illness experience preceding chronic fatigue syndrome: A case control study. *Journal of the Royal College of Physicians of London* 32(1):44-48, 1998.

9. de Rijk AE. Schreurs KM, Bensing JM. General practitioners' attributions of fatigue. *Social Science & Medicine* 47(4):487-496, 1998.

10. Twemlow SW, Bradshaw SL Jr, Coyne L, Lerma BH. Patterns of utilization of medical care and perceptions of the relationship between doctor and patient with chronic illness including chronic fatigue syndrome. *Psychological Reports* 80(2): 643-658, 1997.

11. Ax S, Gregg VH, Jones D. Chronic fatigue syndrome: Sufferers' evaluation of medical support. *Journal of the Royal Society of Medicine* 90(5):250-254, 1997.

12. de Jong LW, Prins JB, Fiselier TJ, Weemaes CM, Meijer-van den Bergh EM, Bleijenberg G. Chronic fatigue syndrome in young persons. *Nederlands Tijdschrift voor Geneeskunde* 141(31):1513-1516, 1997.

13. Libbus MK. Women's beliefs regarding persistent fatigue. *Issues in Mental Health Nursing* 17(6):589-600, 1996.

14. Clements A, Sharpe M, Simkin S, Borrill J, Hawton K. Chronic fatigue syndrome: A qualitative investigation of patients' beliefs about the illness. *Journal of Psychosomatic Research* 42(6):615-624, 1997.

15. Tyrer P, Seivewright H, Seivewright N. Diagnosis of 'ME', which makes an external attribution for fatigue. *Psychological Medicine* 27(2):498-499, 1997.

Immune cell phenotypic distributions

1. Cantor H, Boyse EA. Regulation of cellular and humoral immune responses by T-cell subclasses. *Cold Spring Harbor Symposium on Quantitative Biology* 41:23-32, 1977.

2. Reinherz EL, Schlossmna SF. The characterization and function of human immunoregulatory T lymphocyte subsets. *Immunology Today* 2:6975-6979, 1981.

3. Patarca R, Sandler D, Walling J, Klimas NG, Fletcher MA. Assessment of immune mediator expression levels in biological fluids and cells: A critical appraisal. *Critical Reviews in Oncogenesis* 6(2):117-149, 1995.

4. Calabrese JR, Kling MA, Gold PA. Alterations in immunocompetence during stress, bereavement, and depression: focus on neuroendocrine regulation. *American Journal of Psychiatry* 144:1123-1134, 1987.

5. Fletcher MA, Azen S, Adelberg B et al. Immunophenotyping in a multicenter study: the transfusion safety experience. *Clinical Immunology & Immunopathology* 52:38-47, 1989.

6. Griffin DE. Immunologic abnormalities accompanying acute and chronic viral infections. *Reviews of Infectious Diseases* 13(1):S129-S133, 1991.

7. Klimas N, Patarca R, Perez G et al. Distinctive immune abnormalities in a patient with procainamide-induced lupus and serositis. *American Journal of Medical Sciences* 303(2):1-6, 1992.

8. McAllister CG, Rapaport MH, Pickar D et al. Increased numbers of CD5+ B lymphocytes in schizophrenic patients. *Archives of General Psychiatry* 46:890-894, 1989.

9. Raziuddin S, Elawad ME. Immunoregulatory CD4+CD45R+ suppressor/inducer T lymphocyte subsets and impaired cell-mediated immunity in patients with Down's syndrome. *Clinical and experimental Immunology* 79:67-71, 1990.

10. Villemain F, Chatenoud L, Galinowski A et al. Aberrant T cell-mediated immunity in untreated schizophrenic patients: deficient interleukin-2 production. *American Journal of Psychiatry* 146:609-616, 1989.

11. Herberman RB. Sources of confounding in immunologic data. *Reviews of Infectious Diseases* 13(1):S84-S86, 1991.

12. Lahita RG. Sex hormones and immunity. *Basic and Clinical Immunology.* Stites DP, Stobo JD, Fudenberg HH et al. (eds.), Los Altos, CA, Lange, 1982, pp. 293-294.

13. Malone JL, Simms TE, Gray GC et al. Sources of variability in repeated T-helper lymphocyte counts from human immunodeficiency virus type 1-infected patients: total lymphocyte count fluctuations and diurnal cycle are important. *Journal of Acquired Immune Deficiency Syndromes* 3:144-151, 1990.

14. Martin E, Muler JV, Dionel C. Disappearance of CD4 lymphocyte circadian cycles in HIV-infected patients: early event during asymptomatic infection. *AIDS* 2:133-134, 1988.

15. Patarca R, Sandler D, Walling J, Klimas NG, Fletcher MA. Assessment of immune mediator expression levels in biological fluids and cells: a critical appraisal. *Critical Reviews in Oncogenesis* 6(2):117-149, 1995.

16. Roberts TK, McGregor NR, Dunstan RH, Donohoe M, Murdoch RN, Hope D, Zhang S, Butt HL, Watkins JA, Taylor WG. Immunological and haematological parameters in patients with chronic fatigue syndrome. *Journal of Chronic Fatigue Syndrome* 4(4):51-66, 1998.

17. Schulte PA. Validation of biologic markers for use in research on chronic fatigue syndrome. *Reviews of Infectious Diseases* 13:S87-S89, 1991.

18. Whiteside TL; Cytokine measurements and interpretation in human disease. *Journal of Clinical Immunology* 14:327-339, 1994.

Immunoglobulins

1. Borysiewicz LK, Haworth SJ, Cohen J et al. Epstein-Barr virus—specific immune defects in patients with persistent symptoms following infectious mononucleosis. *Quarterly Journal of Medicine* 58:111-121, 1986.

2. Hamblin TJ, Hussain J, Akbar AN et al. Immunological reason for chronic ill health after infectious mononucleosis. *British Medical Journal* 287:85-88, 1983.

3. Tosato G, Straus S, Henle W et al. Characteristic T-cell dysfunction in patients with chronic active Epstein-Barr virus infection (chronic infectious mononucleosis). *Journal of Immunology* 134:3082-3088, 1985.

4. Buchwald D, Komaroff AL. Review of laboratory findings for patients with chronic fatigue syndrome. *Reviews of Infectious Diseases* 13(1):S12-S18, 1991.

5. Straus SE, Tosato G, Armstrong G et al. Persisting illness and fatigue in adults with evidence of Epstein-Barr virus infection. *Annals of Internal Medicine* 102:7-16, 1985.

6. Klimas N, Salvato F, Morgan R, Fletcher MA. Immunologic abnormalities in chronic fatigue syndrome. *Journal of Clinical Microbiology* 28(6):1403-1410, 1990.

7. Franco K, Kawa HA, Doi S et al. Remarkable depression of CD4+2H4+ T cells in severe chronic active Epstein-Barr virus infection. *Scandinavian Journal of Immunology* 26:769-773, 1987.

8. DuBois RE. Gamma globulin therapy for chronic mononucleosis syndrome. *AIDS Research and Human Retroviruses* 2(1):S191-S195, 1986.

9. Hilgers A, Frank J. Chronic fatigue syndrome: Evaluation of a 30-criteria-score and correlation with immune activation. *Journal of Chronic Fatigue Syndrome* 2(4):35-47, 1996.

10. Jones JF, Ray G, Minnich LL et al. Evidence for active Epstein-Barr virus infection in patients with persistent, unexplained illnesses: elevated anti-early antigen antibodies. *Annals of Internal Medicine* 102:1-7, 1985.

11. Lloyd AR, Wakefield D, Boughton CR et al. Immunological abnormalities in the chronic fatigue syndrome. *Medical Journal of Australia* 151:122-124, 1989.

12. Rasmussen AK, Nielsen AH, Andersen V, Barington T, Bendtzen K, Hansen MB, Nielsen L, Pederson BK, Wiik A. Chronic fatigue syndrome—a controlled cross-sectional study. *The Journal of Rheumatology* 21(8):1527-1531, 1994.

13. Read R, Spickett G, Harvey J et al. IgG1 subclass deficiency in patients with chronic fatigue syndrome. *Lancet* 1:241-242, 1988.

14. Roubalova K, Roubal J, Skopovy P et al. Antibody response to Epstein-Barr virus antigens in patients with chronic viral infection. *Journal of Medical Virology* 25:115-122, 1988.

15. Salit IE. Sporadic postinfectious neuromyasthenia. *Canadian Medical Association Journal* 133:659-663, 1985.

16. Wakefield D, Lloyd A, Brockman A. Immunoglobulin subclass abnormalities in patients with chronic fatigue syndrome. *Journal of Pediatric Infectious Diseases* 9(8):S50-S53, 1990.

17. Gupta S, Vayuvegula B. A comprehensive immunological analysis in chronic fatigue syndrome. *Scandinavian Journal of Immunology* 33(3):319-327, 1991.

18. Lloyd A, Hickie I, Hickie C, Dwyer J, Wakefield D. Cell-mediated immunity in patients with chronic fatigue syndrome, healthy controls and patients with major depression. *Clinical and experimental Immunology* 87(1):76-79, 1992.

19. Mawle AC, Nisenbaum R, Dobbins JG, Gary HE Jr, Stewart JA, Reyes M, Steele L, Schmid DS, Reeves WC. Immune responses associated with chronic fatigue syndrome: A case-control study. *The Journal of Infectious Diseases* 175(1): 136-141, 1997.

20. Natelson BH, LaManca JJ, Denny TN, Vladutiu A, Oleske J, Hill N, Bergen MT, Korn L, Hay J. Immunologic parameters in chronic fatigue syndrome, major depression, and multiple sclerosis. *American Journal of Medicine* 105(3A): 43S-49S, 1998.

21. Peakman M, Deale A, Field R, Mahalingam M, Wessely S. Clinical improvement in chronic fatigue syndrome is not associated with lymphocyte subsets of function or activation. *Clinical Immunology & Immunopathology* 82(1):83-91, 1997.

22. Bates DW, Buchwald D, Lee J, Kith P, Doolittle T, Rutherford C, Churchill WH, Schur PH, Werner M, Wybenga D et al. Clinical laboratory test findings in patients with chronic fatigue syndrome. *Archives of Internal Medicine* 155:97-103, 1995.

23. Komaroff AL, Geiger AM, Wormsley S. IgG subclass deficiencies in chronic fatigue syndrome. *Lancet* 1:1288-1289, 1988.

24. Linde A, Hammarstrom L, Smith CIE. IgG subclass deficiency and chronic fatigue syndrome. *Lancet* 1:885-886, 1988.

25. Lloyd A, Hickie I, Wakefield D et al. A double-blind, placebo-controlled trial of intravenous immunoglobulin therapy in patients with chronic fatigue syndrome. *American Journal of Medicine* 89:561-568, 1990.

26. Peterson PK, Shepard J, Macres M et al. A controlled trial of intravenous immunoglobulin G in chronic fatigue syndrome. *American Journal of Medicine* 89:554-560, 1990.

27. Rowe KS. Double-blind randomized controlled trial to assess the efficacy of intravenous gamma globulin for the management of chronic fatigue syndrome in adolescents. *Journal of Psychiatric Research* 31(1):133-147, 1997.

28. Straus SE. Intravenous immunoglobulin treatment for the chronic fatigue syndrome. *American Journal of Medicine* 89:551-553, 1990.

29. Vollmer-Conna U, Hickie I, Hadzi-Pavlovic D, Tymms K, Wakefield D, Dwyer J, Lloyd A. Intravenous immunoglobulin is ineffective in the treatment of patients with chronic fatigue syndrome. *American Journal of Medicine* 103(1):38-43, 1997.

30. Bennett AL, Fagioli LR, Schur PH, Schacterle RS, Komaroff AL. Immunoglobulin subclass levels in chronic fatigue syndrome. *Journal of Clinical Immunology* 16(6):315-320, 1996.

Inner ear disorders

1. Heller U, Becker EW, Zenner HP, Berg PA. Incidence and clinical relevance of antibodies to phospholipids, serotonin and ganglioside in patients with sudden deafness and progressive inner ear hearing loss. *HNO* 46(6):583-586, 1998.

Interferons (IFNs)

1. Aoki T, Usuda Y, Miyakashi H et al. Low natural syndrome: clinical and immunologic features. *Natural Immunity and Cell Growth Regulation* 6:116-128, 1987.

2. Borysiewicz LK, Haworth SJ, Cohen J et al. Epstein-Barr virus—specific immune defects in patients with persistent symptoms following infectious mononucleosis. *Quarterly Journal of Medicine* 58:111-121, 1986.

3. Buchwald D, Komaroff AL. Review of laboratory findings for patients with chronic fatigue syndrome. *Reviews of Infectious Diseases* 13(1):S12-S18, 1991.

4. Ho-Yen DO, Carrington D, Armstrong AA. Myalgic encephalomyelitis and alpha-interferon. *Lancet* 1:125, 1988.

5. Jones JF, Ray G, Minnich LL et al. Evidence for active Epstein-Barr virus infection in patients with persistent, unexplained illnesses: elevated anti-early antigen antibodies. *Annals of Internal Medicine* 102:1-7, 1985.

6. Lloyd A, Hanna DA, Wakefield D. Interferon and myalgic encephalomyelitis. *Lancet* 1:471, 1988.

7. Straus SE, Tosato G, Armstrong G et al. Persisting illness and fatigue in adults with evidence of Epstein-Barr virus infection. *Annals of Internal Medicine* 102:7-16, 1985.

8. Lever AM, Lewis DM, Bannister BA, Fry M, Berry N. Interferon production in postviral fatigue syndrome. *Lancet* 2(8602):101, 1988.

9. Vojdani A, Ghoneum M, Choppa PC, Magtoto L, Lapp CW. Elevated apoptotic cell population in patients with chronic fatigue syndrome: The pivotal role of protein kinase RNA. *Journal of Internal Medicine* 242(6):465-478, 1997.

10. Linde A, Andersson B, Svenson SB, Ahrne H, Carlsson M, Forsberg P, Hugo H, Karstop A, Lenkei R, Lindwall A et al. Serum levels of lymphokines and soluble cellular receptors in primary EBV infection and in patients with chronic fatigue syndrome. *The Journal of Infectious Diseases* 165:994-1000, 1992.

11. Straus SE, Dale JK, Peter JB, Dinarello CA. Circulating lymphokine levels in the chronic fatigue syndrome. *The Journal of Infectious Diseases* 160(6):1085-1086, 1989.

12. Dalakas MC, Mock V, Hawkins MJ. Fatigue: Definitions, mechanisms, and paradigms for study. *Seminars in Oncology* 25(1 Suppl 1):48-53, 1998.

13. Jones TH, Wadler S, Hupart KH. Endocrine-mediated mechanisms of fatigue during treatment with interferon-alpha. *Seminars in Oncology* 25(1 Suppl 1):54-63, 1998.

14. Davis JM, Weaver JA, Kohut ML, Colbert LH, Ghaffar A, Mayer EP. Immune system activation and fatigue during treadmill running: Role of interferon. *Medicine & Science in Sports & Exercise* 30(6):863-868, 1998.

15. Zlotnick A, Shimonkewitz P, Gefter ML et al. Characterization of the gamma interferon-mediated induction of antigen-presenting ability in P388D cells. *Journal of Immunology* 131:2814-2820, 1983.

16. Targan S, Stebbing N. In vitro interactions of purified cloned human interferons on NK cells: enhanced activation. *Journal of Immunology* 129:934-935, 1982.

17. Knop J, Stremer R, Nauman C et al. Interferon inhibits the suppressor T-cell response of delayed hypersensitivity. *Nature* 296:757-759, 1982.

18. Klimas N, Salvato F, Morgan R, Fletcher MA. Immunologic abnormalities in chronic fatigue syndrome. *Journal of Clinical Microbiology* 28(6):1403-1410, 1990.

19. Visser J, Blauw B, Hinloopen B, Brommer E, de Kloet ER, Kluft C, Nagelkerken L. CD4 T lymphocytes from patients with chronic fatigue syndrome have decreased interferon-gamma production and increased sensitivity to dexamethasone. *The Journal of Infectious Diseases* 177(2):451-454, 1998.

20. Lloyd A, Hickie I, Hickie C, Dwyer J, Wakefield D. Cell-mediated immunity in patients with chronic fatigue syndrome, healthy controls and patients with major depression. *Clinical and experimental Immunology* 87(1):76-79, 1992.

21. Peakman M, Deale A, Field R, Mahalingam M, Wessely S. Clinical improvement in chronic fatigue syndrome is not associated with lymphocyte subsets of function or activation. *Clinical Immunology & Immunopathology* 82(1):83-91, 1997.

Interleukin-1 (IL-1) and soluble IL-1 receptors

1. Dinarello CA. Interleukin-1 and interleukin-1 antagonism. *Blood* 77(8):1627-1652, 1991.

2. Platanias LC, Vogelzang NJ. Interleukin-1: Biology, pathophysiology, and clinical prospects. *American Journal of Medicine* 89:621-629, 1990.

3. Patarca R, Lugtendorf S, Antoni M, Klimas NG, Fletcher MA. Dysregulated expression of tumor necrosis factor in the chronic fatigue immune dysfunction syndrome: Interrelations with cellular sources and patterns of soluble immune mediator expression. *Clinical Infectious Diseases* 18:S147-S153, 1994.

4. Linde A, Andersson B, Svenson SB, Ahrne H, Carlsson M, Forsberg P, Hugo H, Karstop A, Lenkei R, Lindwall A et al. Serum levels of lymphokines and soluble cellular receptors in primary EBV infection and in patients with chronic fatigue syndrome. *The Journal of Infectious Diseases* 165:994-1000, 1992.

5. Lloyd A, Hickie I, Hickie C, Dwyer J, Wakefield D. Cell-mediated immunity in patients with chronic fatigue syndrome, healthy controls and patients with major depression. *Clinical and experimental Immunology* 87(1):76-79, 1992.

6. Peakman M, Deale A, Field R, Mahalingam M, Wessely S. Clinical improvement in chronic fatigue syndrome is not associated with lymphocyte subsets of function or activation. *Clinical Immunology & Immunopathology* 82(1):83-91, 1997.

7. Rasmussen AK, Nielsen AH, Andersen V, Barington T, Bendtzen K, Hansen MB, Nielsen L, Pederson BK, Wiik A. Chronic fatigue syndrome—a controlled cross-sectional study. *The Journal of Rheumatology* 21(8):1527-1531, 1994.

8. Morte S, Castilla A, Civeira MP, Serrano M, Prieto J. Production of interleukin-1 by peripheral blood mononuclear cells in patients with chronic fatigue syndrome. *The Journal of Infectious Diseases* 159:362, 1989.

9. Straus SE, Dale JK, Peter JB, Dinarello CA. Circulating lymphokine levels in the chronic fatigue syndrome. *The Journal of Infectious Diseases* 160(6): 1085-1086, 1989.

10. Arnason BGW. Nervous system—immune system communication. *Reviews of Infectious Diseases* 13(1):S134-S137, 1991.

11. Berkenbosch F, Van Oers J, Del Rey A et al. Corticotropin-releasing factor-producing neurons in the RT activated by interleukin-1. *Science* 238:524-526, 1987.

12. Besedorsky H, Del Rey A, Sorkin E et al. Immunoregulatory feedback between interleukin-1 and glucocorticoid hormones. *Science* 233:652-654, 1986.

13. Sapolsky R, Rivier C, Yamamoto G et al. Interleukin-1 stimulates the secretion of hypothalamic corticotropin-releasing factor. *Science* 233:522-524, 1987.

14. Bernton EW, Beach J, Holaday JW et al. Release of multiple hormones by a direct action of interleukin-1 on pituitary cells. *Science* 238:519-521, 1987.

15. Rettori V, Gimeno MF, Karara A et al. Interleukin-1a inhibits protaglandin E_2 release to suppress pulsatile release of luteinizing hormone but not follicle-stimulating hormone. *Proceedings of the National Academy of Sciences of the United States of America* 88:2763-2767, 1991.

16. Shoham S, Davenne D, Cady AB et al. Recombinant tumor necrosis factor and interleukin-1 enhance slow wave sleep. *American Journal of Physiology* 253:R142-R149, 1987.

17. Holmes GP, Kaplan JE, Gantz NM et al. Chronic fatigue syndrome: A working case definition. *Annals of Internal Medicine* 108:387-389, 1988.

18. Moldovsky H. Nonrestorative sleep and symptoms after a febrile illness in patients with fibrosis and chronic fatigue syndrome. *The Journal of Rheumatology* 16(19):150-153, 1989.

19. Dejana E, Brenario F, Erroi A et al. Modulation of endothelial cell function by different molecular species of interleukin-1. *Blood* 69:635-699, 1987.

20. Caverzasio J, Rizzoli R, Dayer JM. Interleukin-1 decreases renal sodium reabsorption: Possible mechanisms of endotoxin-induced natriuresis. *American Journal of Physiology* 252:943-6, 1987.

21. Gulick T, Chung MK, Pieper SJ et al. Interleukin-1 and tumor necrosis factor inhibit cardiac myocyte beta-adrenergic responsiveness. *Proceedings of the National Academy of Sciences of the United States of America* 86:6753-6757, 1989.

22. Cannon JG, Angel JB, Abad LW, Vannier E, Mileno MD, Fagioli L, Wolff SM, Komaroff AL. Interleukin-1 beta, interleukin-1 receptor antagonist, and soluble interleukin-1 receptor type II secretion in chronic fatigue syndrome. *Journal of Clinical Immunology* 17(3):253-261, 1997.

23. Swanink CM, Vercoulen JH, Galama JM, Roos MT, Meyaard L, van der Ven-Jongekrijg J, de Nijs R, Bleijenberg G, Fennis JF, Miedema F, van der Meer JW. Lymphocyte subsets, apoptosis, and cytokines in patients with chronic fatigue syndrome. *The Journal of Infectious Diseases* 173(2):460-463, 1996.

Interleukin-2 (IL-2) and soluble IL-2 receptor

1. Watson J, Mochizuki D. Interleukin-2: A class of T-cell growth factor. *Inmmunological Reviews* 51:257-278, 1980.

2. Fletcher M, Goldstein AL. Recent advances in the understanding of the biochemistry and clinical pharmacology of interelukin-2. *Lymphokine Research* 1:45-57, 1987.

3. Morgan DA, Ruscetti FW, Gallo RC. Selective in vitro growth of T lymphocytes from normal human bone marrows. *Science* 193:1007-1008, 1976.

4. Malkovsky M, Loveland B, Noth M et al. Recombinant interleukin-2 directly augments the cytotoxicity of human monocytes. *Nature* 325:262-265, 1987.

5. Tsudo M, Ichiyama T, Uchino H. Expression of Tac antigen on activated normal human B cells. *Journal of Experimental Medicine* 160:612-617, 1984.

6. Cheney PR, Dorman SE, Bell DS. Interleukin-2 and the chronic fatigue syndrome. *Annals of Internal Medicine* 110(4):321, 1989.

7. Gold D, Bowden R, Sixbey J et al. Chronic fatigue. A prospective clinical and virologic study. *JAMA* 264:48-53, 1990.

8. Kibler R, Lucas DO, Hicks M et al. Immune function in chronic active Epstein-Barr virus infection. *Journal of Clinical Immunology* 5:46-54, 1985.

9. Linde A, Andersson B, Svenson SB, Ahrne H, Carlsson M, Forsberg P, Hugo H, Karstop A, Lenkei R, Lindwall A et al. Serum levels of lymphokines and soluble cellular receptors in primary EBV infection and in patients with chronic fatigue syndrome. *The Journal of Infectious Diseases* 165:994-1000, 1992.

10. Patarca R, Lugtendorf S, Antoni M, Klimas NG, Fletcher MA. Dysregulated expression of tumor necrosis factor in the chronic fatigue immune dysfunction syndrome: Interrelations with cellular sources and patterns of soluble immune mediator expression. *Clinical Infectious Diseases* 18:S147-S153, 1994.

11. Straus SE, Dale JK, Peter JB, Dinarello CA. Circulating lymphokine levels in the chronic fatigue syndrome. *The Journal of Infectious Diseases* 160(6): 1085-1086, 1989.

12. Rasmussen AK, Nielsen AH, Andersen V, Barington T, Bendtzen K, Hansen MB, Nielsen L, Pederson BK, Wiik A. Chronic fatigue syndrome—a controlled cross-sectional study. *The Journal of Rheumatology* 21(8):1527-1531, 1994.

13. Cohen N, Stempel C, Colombe B et al. Soluble interleukin-2 receptor: Detection and potential role in organ transplantation. *Clinical Immunology Newsletter* 10(12):175, 1990.

14. Pui CH. Serum interleukin-2 receptor: Clinical and biological implications. *Leukemia* 3(5):323-327, 1989.

Interleukin-4 (IL-4)

1. Paul WE, Ohara J. B-cell stimulatory factor-1/interleukin-4. *Annual Reviews of Immunology* 5:429-459, 1987.

2. Kuehn R, Rajewsky K, Mueller W. Generation and analysis of interleukin-4 deficient mice. *Science* 254:713-716, 1991.

3. Visser J, Blauw B, Hinloopen B, Brommer E, de Kloet ER, Kluft C, Nagelkerken L. CD4 T lymphocytes from patients with chronic fatigue syndrome have decreased interferon-gamma production and increased sensitivity to dexamethasone. *The Journal of Infectious Diseases* 177(2):451-454, 1998.

Interleukin-6 (IL-6) and soluble IL-6 receptor

1. Mizel SB. The interleukins. *FASEB Journal* 3:2379-2388, 1989.
2. Van Snick J. Interleukin-6: An overview. *Annual Reviews of Immunology* 8:253-278, 1990.
3. Gupta S, Aggarwal S, See D, Starr A. Cytokine production by adherent and non-adherent mononuclear cells in chronic fatigue syndrome. *Journal of Psychiatric Research* 31(1):149-156, 1997.
4. Buchwald D, Wener MH, Pearlman T, Kith P. Markers of inflammation and immune activation in chronic fatigue and chronic fatigue syndrome. *The Journal of Rheumatology* 24(2):372-6, 1997.
5. Chao CC, Gallagher M, Phair J, Peterson PK. Serum neopterin and interleukin-6 levels in chronic fatigue syndrome. *The Journal of Infectious Diseases* 162:1412-1413, 1990.
6. Chao CC, Janoff EN, Hu S, Thomas K, Gallagher M, Tsang M, Peterson PK. Altered cytokine release in peripheral blood mononuclear cell cultures from patients with the chronic fatigue syndrome. *Cytokine* 3:292-298, 1991.
7. Linde A, Andersson B, Svenson SB, Ahrne H, Carlsson M, Forsberg P, Hugo H, Karstop A, Lenkei R, Lindwall A et al. Serum levels of lymphokines and soluble cellular receptors in primary EBV infection and in patients with chronic fatigue syndrome. *The Journal of Infectious Diseases* 165:994-1000, 1992.
8. Lloyd A, Hickie I, Hickie C, Dwyer J, Wakefield D. Cell-mediated immunity in patients with chronic fatigue syndrome, healthy controls and patients with major depression. *Clinical and experimental Immunology* 87(1):76-79, 1992.
9. Patarca R, Lugtendorf S, Antoni M, Klimas NG, Fletcher MA. Dysregulated expression of tumor necrosis factor in the chronic fatigue immune dysfunction syndrome: Interrelations with cellular sources and patterns of soluble immune mediator expression. *Clinical Infectious Diseases* 18:S147-S153, 1994.
10. Peakman M, Deale A, Field R, Mahalingam M, Wessely S. Clinical improvement in chronic fatigue syndrome is not associated with lymphocyte subsets of function or activation. *Clinical Immunology & Immunopathology* 82(1):83-91, 1997.
11. Penttila IA, Harris RJ, Storm P, Haynes D, Worswick DA, Marmion BP. Cytokine dysregulation in the post–Q-fever syndrome. *Quarterly Journal of Medicine* 91(8):549-560, 1998.
12. Patarca R, Klimas NG, Garcia MN, Pons H, Fletcher MA. Dysregulated expression of soluble immune mediator receptors in a subset of patients with chronic fatigue syndrome: Categorization of patients by immune status. *Journal of Chronic Fatigue Syndrome* 1:79-94, 1995.

Interleukin-10 (IL-10)

1. Gupta S, Aggarwal S, See D, Starr A. Cytokine production by adherent and non-adherent mononuclear cells in chronic fatigue syndrome. *Journal of Psychiatric Research* 31(1):149-156, 1997.

Interstitial cystitis

1. Korszun A, Papadopoulos E, Demitrack M, Engleberg C, Crofford L. The relationship between temporomandibular disorders and stress-associated syndromes. *Oral Surgery, Oral Medicine, Oral Pathology, Oral Radiology, & Endodontics* 86(4):416-20, 1998.

Lead poisoning

1. Mesch U, Lowenthal RM, Coleman D. Lead poisoning masquerading as chronic fatigue syndrome. *Lancet* 347(9009):1193, 1996.

Lentiviruses

1. Holmes MJ, Diack DS, Easingwood A, Cross JP, Carlisle B. Electron microscope immunocytological profiles in chronic fatigue syndrome. *Journal of Psychiatric Research* 31(1):115-22, 1997.

Low cysteine-glutathione syndrome

1. Droge W, Holm E. Role of cysteine and glutathione in HIV infection and other diseases associated with muscle wasting and immunological dysfunction. *FASEB Journal* 11(13):1077-1089, 1997.

Lymphocytes

1. Reinherz EL, Schlossman SF. The characterization and function of human immunoregulatory T lymphocyte subsets. *Immunology Today* 2:6975-6979, 1981.
2. Straus SE, Tosato G, Armstrong G et al. Persisting illness and fatigue in adults with evidence of Epstein-Barr virus infection. *Annals of Internal Medicine* 102:7-16, 1985.
3. Jones J. Serologic and immunologic responses in chronic fatigue syndrome with emphasis on the Epstein-Barr virus. *Reviews of Infectious Diseases* 13(1): S26-S31, 1991.
4. Jones JF, Straus SE. Chronic Epstein-Barr virus infection. *Annual Revue of Medicine* 38:195-209, 1987.
5. Jones JF, Ray G, Minnich LL et al. Evidence for active Epstein-Barr virus infection in patients with persistent, unexplained illnesses: elevated anti-early antigen antibodies. *Annals of Internal Medicine* 102:1-7, 1985.
6. Borysiewicz LK, Haworth SJ, Cohen J et al. Epstein-Barr virus—specific immune defects in patients with persistent symptoms following infectious mononucleosis. *Quarterly Journal of Medicine* 58:111-121, 1986.

7. Gupta S, Vayuvegula B. A comprehensive immunological analysis in chronic fatigue syndrome. *Scandinavian Journal of Immunology* 33(3):319-327, 1991.

8. Landay AL, Jessop C, Lennette ET, Levy JA. Chronic fatigue syndrome: clinical condition associated with immune activation. *Lancet* 338:707-712, 1991.

9. Lloyd A, Hickie I, Hickie C, Dwyer J, Wakefield D. Cell-mediated immunity in patients with chronic fatigue syndrome, healthy controls and patients with major depression. *Clinical and experimental Immunology* 87(1):76-79, 1992.

10. Tirelli U, Marotta G, Improta S, Pinto A. Immunological abnormalities in patients with chronic fatigue syndrome. *Scandinavian Journal of Immunology* 40(6):601-608, 1994.

11. Lloyd AR, Wakefield D, Boughton CR et al. Immunological abnormalities in the chronic fatigue syndrome. *Medical Journal of Australia* 151:122-124, 1989.

12. Buchwald D, Komaroff AL. Review of laboratory findings for patients with chronic fatigue syndrome. *Reviews of Infectious Diseases* 13(1):S12-S18, 1991.

13. Klimas N, Salvato F, Morgan R, Fletcher MA. Immunologic abnormalities in chronic fatigue syndrome. *Journal of Clinical Microbiology* 28(6):1403-1410, 1990.

14. Aoki T, Usuda Y, Miyakashi H et al. Low natural syndrome: Clinical and immunologic features. *Natural Immunity and Cell Growth Regulation* 6:116-128, 1987.

15. DuBois RE. Gamma globulin therapy for chronic mononucleosis syndrome. *AIDS Research and Human Retroviruses* 2(1):S191-S195, 1986.

16. Linde A, Andersson B, Svenson SB, Ahrne H, Carlsson M, Forsberg P, Hugo H, Karstop A, Lenkei R, Lindwall A et al. Serum levels of lymphokines and soluble cellular receptors in primary EBV infection and in patients with chronic fatigue syndrome. *The Journal of Infectious Diseases* 165:994-1000, 1992.

17. Mawle AC, Nisenbaum R, Dobbins JG, Gary HE Jr, Stewart JA, Reyes M, Steele L, Schmid DS, Reeves WC. Immune responses associated with chronic fatigue syndrome: A case-control study. *The Journal of Infectious Diseases* 175(1):136-141, 1997.

18. Patarca R, Goodkin K, Fletcher MA. Cryopreservation of peripheral blood mononuclear cells. *Manual of Clinical Laboratory Immunology,* Rose NR, de Macario EC, Folds JD, Lane HC, Nakamura RM (eds.), pp. 281-286, 1995.

19. Sandman CA, Barron JL, Nackoul KA, Fidler PL, Goldstein J. Is there a chronic fatigue syndrome (CFS) dementia? *The Clinical and Scientific Basis of Myalgic Encephalomyelitis/Chronic Fatigue Syndrome,* Hyde B, Levine P, Goldstein J (eds.), Nightingale Research Foundation. Ottawa Canada, 1992, pp. 467-479.

20. Morimoto C, Letvin NL, Distaso JA et al. The isolation and characterization of the human suppressor inducer T-cell subset. *Journal of Immunology* 134: 1508-1512, 1985.

21. Natelson BH, LaManca JJ, Denny TN, Vladutiu A, Oleske J, Hill N, Bergen MT, Korn L, Hay J. Immunologic parameters in chronic fatigue syndrome, major depression, and multiple sclerosis. *American Journal of Medicine* 105(3A): 43S-49S, 1998.

22. Franco K, Kawa HA, Doi S et al. Remarkable depression of CD4+2H4+ T cells in severe chronic active Epstein-Barr virus infection. *Scandinavian Journal of Immunology* 26:769-773, 1987.

23. Alpert S, Kloide J, Takada S et al. T-cell regulatory disturbances in the rheumatic diseases. *Rheumatic Diseases Clinics of North America* 13(3):431-435, 1987.

24. Emery P, Gently KC, Mackay IR et al. Deficiency of the suppressor inducer subset of T lymphocytes in rheumatoid arthritis. *Arthitis & Rheumatism* 30: 849-856, 1987.

25. Klimas N, Patarca R, Perez G et al. Distinctive immune abnormalities in a patient with procainamide-induced lupus and serositis. *The American Journal of Medical Sciences* 303(2):1-6, 1992.

26. Sato K, Miyasaka N, Yamaoka K et al. Quantitative defect of CD4+2H4+ cells in systemic lupus erythematosus and Sjögren's syndrome. *Arthritis & Rheumatism* 30:1407-1411, 1987.

27. Sobel RA, Hafler DA, Castro EE et al. The 2H4 (CD45R) antigen is selectively decreased in multiple sclerosis lesions. *Journal of Immunology* 140: 2210-2214, 1988.

28. Barker E, Fujimura SF, Fadem MB, Landay AL, Levy JA. Immunologic abnormalities associated with chronic fatigue syndrome. *Clinical Infectious Diseases* 18(Supp 1):S136-S141, 1994.

29. Hassan IS, Bannister BA, Akbar A, Weir W, Bofill M. A study of the immunology of the chronic fatigue syndrome: Correlation of immunologic markers to health dysfunction. *Clinical Immunology & Immunopathology* 87(1):60-67, 1998.

30. Swanink CM, Vercoulen JH, Galama JM, Roos MT, Meyaard L, van der Ven-Jongekrijg J, de Nijs R, Bleijenberg G, Fennis JF, Miedema F, van der Meer JW. Lymphocyte subsets, apoptosis, and cytokines in patients with chronic fatigue syndrome. *The Journal of Infectious Diseases* 173(2):460-463, 1996.

31. Peakman M, Deale A, Field R, Mahalingam M, Wessely S. Clinical improvement in chronic fatigue syndrome is not associated with lymphocyte subsets of function or activation. *Clinical Immunology & Immunopathology* 82(1):83-91, 1997.

32. Alviggi L, Johnson C, Hopkins PJ et al. Pathogenesis of insulin-dependent diabetes: a role for activated T lymphocytes. *Lancet* 2:4-6, 1984.

33. Canonina GW, Bagnasco M, Corte G et al. Circulating T lymphocytes in Hashimoto's disease: imbalance of subsets and presence of activated cells. *Clinical Immunology & Immunopathology* 23:616-625, 1982.

34. Jackson RA, Haynes BF, Burch WM et al. Ia+ T cells in new onset Grave's disease. *Journal of Clinical Endocrinology and Metabolism* 59:187-190, 1984.

35. Koide J. Functional property of Ia-positive T cells in peripheral blood from patients with systemic lupus erythematosus. *Scandinavian Journal of Immunology* 22:577-584, 1985.

36. Rabinowe SL, Jackson RA, Dluhy RG et al. Ia-positive T lymphocytes in recently diagnosed idiopathic Addison's disease. *American Journal of Medicine* 77:597-601, 1984.

37. Behan PO, Behan WHM, Bell EJ. The postviral fatigue syndrome—An analysis of the findings in 50 cases. *Journal of Infectious Diseases* 10:211-22, 1985.

38. Lloyd AR, Wakefield D, Boughton CR et al. Immunological abnormalities in the chronic fatigue syndrome. *Medical Journal of Australia* 151:122-124, 1989.

39. Lloyd A, Hickie I, Hickie C, Dwyer J, Wakefield D. Cell-mediated immunity in patients with chronic fatigue syndrome, healthy controls and patients with major depression. *Clinical and experimental Immunology* 87(1):76-79, 1992.

40. Straus SE, Tosato G, Armstrong G et al. Persisting illness and fatigue in adults with evidence of Epstein-Barr virus infection. *Annals of Internal Medicine* 102:7-16, 1985.

41. Tobi M, Morag A, Ravid Z et al. Prolonged atypical illness associated with serological evidence of persistent Epstein-Barr infection. *Lancet* 1:61-64, 1982.

42. Roberts TK, McGregor NR, Dunstan RH, Donohoe M, Murdoch RN, Hope D, Zhang S, Butt HL, Watkins JA, Taylor WG. Immunological and haematological parameters in patients with chronic fatigue syndrome. *Journal of Chronic Fatigue Syndrome* 4(4):51-66, 1998.

43. Subira ML, Castilla A, Civeira MP et al. Deficient display of CD3 on lymphocytes of patients with chronic fatigue syndrome. *The Journal of Infectious Diseases* 160:165-166, 1989.

44. Casali P, Notkins AL. CD5+ B lymphocytes, polyreactive antibodies and the human B-cell repertoire. *Immunology Today* 10:364-368, 1989.

45. Olson GB, Kanaan MN, Gersuk GM et al. Correlation between allergy and persistent Epstein-Barr virus infections in chronic active Epstein-Barr virus infected patients. *Journal of Allergy and Clinical Immunology* 78:308-314, 1986.

46. Olson GB, Kanaan MN, Kelley LM et al. Specific allergen-induced Epstein-Barr nuclear antigen-positive B cells from patients with chronic active Epstein-Barr virus infections. *Journal of Allergy Clinical Immunology* 78:315-320, 1986.

Monoamine oxidase (MAO) inhibitors

1. Natelson BH, Cheu J, Pareja J, Ellis SP, Policastro T, Findley TW. Randomized, double-blind, controlled placebo-phase in trial of low dose phenelzine in the chronic fatigue syndrome. *Psychopharmacology* 124(3):226-230, 1996.

2. Natelson BH, Cheu J, Hill N, Bergen M, Korn L, Denny T, Dahl K. Single-blind, placebo phase-in trial of two escalating doses of selegeline in the chronic fatigue syndrome. *Neuropsychobiology* 37(3):150-154, 1998.

Monocytes

1. Prieto J, Subira ML, Castilla A et al. Naloxone-reversible monocyte dysfunction in patients with chronic fatigue syndrome. *Scandinavian Journal of Immunology* 30:13-20, 1989.

2. Gupta S, Vayuvegula B. A comprehensive immunological analysis in chronic fatigue syndrome. *Scandinavian Journal of Immunology* 33(3):319-327, 1991.

3. Barker E, Fujimura SF, Fadem MB, Landay AL, Levy JA. Immunologic abnormalities associated with chronic fatigue syndrome. *Clinical Infectious Diseases* 18(supp 1):S136-S141, 1994.

Multiple chemical sensitivity (MCS) syndrome

1. Bell IR, Baldwin CM, Schwartz GE. Illness from low levels of environmental chemicals: Relevance to chronic fatigue syndrome and fibromyalgia. *American Journal of Medicine* 105(3A):74S-82S, 1998.
2. Weiss B. Neurobehavioral properties of chemical sensitivity syndromes. *Neurotoxicology* 19(2):259-268, 1998.
3. Fiedler N, Kipen HM, DeLuca J, Kelly-McNeil K, Natelson B. A controlled comparison of multiple chemical sensitivities and chronic fatigue syndrome. *Psychosomatic Medicine* 58(1):38-49, 1996.
4. Lohmann K, Prohl A, Schwarz E. Multiple chemical sensitivity disorder in patients with neurotoxic illnesses. *Gesundheitswesen* 58(6):322-331, 1996.
5. Gibson PR, Cheavens J, Warren ML. Social support in persons with self-reported sensitivity to chemicals. *Research in Nursing & Health* 21(2):103-115, 1998.

Multiple sclerosis (MS)

1. Taylor RS. Multiple sclerosis potpourri. Paroxysmal symptoms, seizures, fatigue, pregnancy, and more. *Physical Medicine & Rehabilitation Clinics of North America* 9(3):551-559, 1998.
2. Dulli D, Schutta H. Fatigue in MS. *Neurology* 47(5):1351, 1996; Poser CM. Fatigue in MS. *Neurology* 47(5):1351, 1996.
3. Bergamaschi R, Romani A, Versino M, Poli R, Cosi V. Clinical aspects of fatigue in multiple sclerosis. *Functional Neurology* 12(5):247-251, 1997.
4. Ford H, Trigwell P, Johnson M. The nature of fatigue in multiple sclerosis. *Journal of Psychosomatic Research* 45:33-38, 1998.
5. Tola MA, Yugueros MI, Fernandez-Buey N, Fernandez-Herranz R. Impact of fatigue in multiple sclerosis: Study of a population-based series in Valladolid. *Revista de Neurologia* 26(154):930-933, 1998.
6. Krupp LB, Pollina DA. Mechanisms and management of fatigue in progressive neurological disorders. *Current Opinions in Neurology* 9(6):456-460, 1996.
7. Stuifbergen AK, Rogers S. The experience of fatigue and strategies of self-care among persons with multiple sclerosis. *Applied Nursing Research* 10(1):2-10, 1997.
8. Vercoulen JH, Hommes OR, Swanink CM, Jongen PJ, Fennis JF, Galama JM, van der Meer JW, Bleijenberg G. The measurement of fatigue in patients with multiple sclerosis. A multidimensional comparison with patients with chronic fatigue syndrome and healthy subjects. *Archives of Neurology* 53(7):642-649, 1996.
9. Tantucci C, Massucci M, Piperno R, Grassi V, Sorbini CA. Energy cost of exercise in multiple sclerosis patients with low degree of disability. *Multiple Sclerosis* 2(3):161-167, 1996.

10. Latash M, Kalugina E, Nicholas J, Orpett C, Stefoski D, Davis F. Myogenic and central neurogenic factors in fatigue in multiple sclerosis. *Multiple Sclerosis* 1(4):236-241, 1996.

11. Fukazawa T, Sasaki H, Kikuchi S, Hamada T, Tashiro K. Serum carnitine and disabling fatigue in multiple sclerosis. *Psychiatry & Clinical Neuroscience* 50(6):323-325, 1996.

12. Sheean GL, Murray NM, Rothwell JC, Miller DH, Thompson AJ. An electrophysiological study of the mechanism of fatigue in multiple sclerosis. *Brain* 120(Pt 2):299-315, 1997.

13. Wei T, Lightman SL. The neuroendocrine axis in patients with multiple sclerosis. *Brain* 120(Pt 6):1067-1076, 1997.

14. Iriarte J, Carreno M, de Castro P. Fatigue and functional system involvement in multiple sclerosis. *Neurologia* 11(6):210-215, 1996.

15. Djaldetti R, Ziv I, Achiron A, Melamed E. Fatigue in multiple sclerosis compared with chronic fatigue syndrome: A quantitative assessment. *Neurology* 46(3):632-5, 1996.

16. Taylor A, Taylor RS. Neuropsychologic aspects of multiple sclerosis. *Physical Medicine & Rehabilitation Clinics of North America* 9(3):643-657, 1998.

17. Deatrick JA, Brennan D, Cameron ME. Mothers with multiple sclerosis and their children: Effects of fatigue and exacerbations on maternal support. *Nursing Research* 47(4):205-210, 1998.

18. Rosenblum D, Saffir M. Therapeutic and symptomatic treatment of multiple sclerosis. *Physical Medicine & Rehabilitation Clinics of North America* 9(3):587-601, 1998.

19. Neilley LK, Goodin DS, Goodkin DE, Hauser SL. Side effect profile of interferon beta-1b in MS: Results of an open label trial. *Neurology* 46(2):552-554, 1996.

20. Metz L. Multiple sclerosis: symptomatic therapies. *Seminars in Neurology* 18(3):389-395, 1998.

21. Consroe P, Musty R, Rein J, Tillery W, Pertwee R. The perceived effects of smoked cannabis on patients with multiple sclerosis. *European Neurology* 38(1):44-48, 1997.

22. Sheean GL, Murray NM, Rothwell JC, Miller DH, Thompson AJ. An openlabelled clinical and electrophysiological study of 3,4 diaminopyridine in the treatment of fatigue in multiple sclerosis. *Brain* 121(Pt 5):967-975, 1998.

23. LaBan MM, Martin T, Pechur J, Sarnacki S. Physical and occupational therapy in the treatment of patients with multiple sclerosis. *Physical Medicine & Rehabilitation Clinics of North America* 9(3):603-614, 1998.

24. Di Fabio RP, Soderberg J, Choi T, Hansen CR, Schapiro RT. Extended outpatient rehabilitation: Its influence on symptom frequency, fatigue, and functional status for persons with progressive multiple sclerosis. *Archives of Physical Medicine & Rehabilitation* 79(2):141-146, 1998.

Muscle physiology

1. Vecchiet L, Montanari G, Pizzigallo E, Iezzi S, de Bigontina P, Dragani L, Vecchiet J, Giamberardino MA. Sensory characterization of somatic parietal tissues in humans with chronic fatigue syndrome. *Neuroscience Letters* 208(2):117-120, 1996.
2. Lodi R, Taylor DJ, Radda GK. Chronic fatigue syndrome and skeletal muscle mitochondrial function. *Muscle & Nerve* 20(6):765-766, 1997.
3. Lane RJ, Barrett MC, Taylor DJ, Kemp GJ, Lodi R. Heterogeneity in chronic fatigue syndrome: Evidence from magnetic resonance spectroscopy of muscle. *Neuromuscular Disorders* 8(3-4):204-209, 1998.
4. Lane RJ, Barrett MC, Woodrow D, Moss J, Fletcher R, Archard LC. Muscle fibre characteristics and lactate responses to exercise in chronic fatigue syndrome. *Journal of Neurology, Neurosurgery & Psychiatry* 64(3):362-367, 1998.
5. McCully KK, Natelson BH, Iotti S, Sisto S, Leigh JS Jr. Reduced oxidative muscle metabolism in chronic fatigue syndrome. *Muscle & Nerve* 19(5):621-625, 1996.
6. Bowman MA, Kirk JK, Michielutte R, Preisser JS. Use of amantadine for chronic fatigue syndrome. *Archives of Internal Medicine* 157(11):1264-1265, 1997.
7. Plioplys AV, Plioplys S. Amantadine and L-carnitine treatment of chronic fatigue syndrome. *Neuropsychobiology* 35(1):16-23, 1997.

Mycoplasma

1. Choppa PC, Vojdani A, Tagle C, Andrin R, Magtoto L. Multiplex PCR for the detection of Mycoplasma fermentans, M. hominis and M. penetrans in cell cultures and blood samples of patients with chronic fatigue syndrome. *Molecular & Cellular Probes* 12(5):301-308, 1998.

Natural killer (NK) cells

1. Patarca R, Fletcher MA, Podack ER. Cytolytic cell functions. *Manual of Clinical Laboratory Immunology.* Rose NR, de Macario EC, Folds JD, Lane HC, Nakamura RM (eds.), Washington DC, American Society for Microbiology, 1995, pp 296-303.
2. Klimas N, Salvato F, Morgan R, Fletcher MA. Immunologic abnormalities in chronic fatigue syndrome. *Journal of Clinical Microbiology* 28(6):1403-1410, 1990.
3. Morrison LJ, Behan WH, Behan PO. Changes in natural killer cell phenotype in patients with post-viral fatigue syndrome. *Clinical and experimental Immunology* 83:441-446, 1991.
4. Peakman M, Deale A, Field R, Mahalingam M, Wessely S. Clinical improvement in chronic fatigue syndrome is not associated with lymphocyte subsets of function or activation. *Clinical Immunology & Immunopathology* 82(1):83-91, 1997.

5. Tirelli U, Marotta G, Improta S, Pinto A. Immunological abnormalities in patients with chronic fatigue syndrome. *Scandinavian Journal of Immunology* 40(6):601-608, 1994.

6. Barker E, Fujimura SF, Fadem MB, Landay AL, Levy JA. Immunologic abnormalities associated with chronic fatigue syndrome. *Clinical Infectious Diseases* 18(Supp 1):S136-S141, 1994.

7. Landay AL, Jessop C, Lennette ET, Levy JA. Chronic fatigue syndrome: clinical condition associated with immune activation. *Lancet* 338:707-712, 1991.

8. Lloyd A, Hickie I, Hickie C, Dwyer J, Wakefield D. Cell-mediated immunity in patients with chronic fatigue syndrome, healthy controls and patients with major depression. *Clinical and experimental Immunology* 87(1):76-79, 1992.

9. Natelson BH, LaManca JJ, Denny TN, Vladutiu A, Oleske J, Hill N, Bergen MT, Korn L, Hay J. Immunologic parameters in chronic fatigue syndrome, major depression, and multiple sclerosis. *American Journal of Medicine* 105(3A): 43S-49S, 1998.

10. Masuda A, Nozoe SI, Matsuyama T, Tanaka H. Psychobehavioral and immunological characteristics of adult people with chronic fatigue and patients with chronic fatigue syndrome. *Psychosomatic Medicine* 56(6):516-518, 1994.

11. Gupta S, Vayuvegula B. A comprehensive immunological analysis in chronic fatigue syndrome. *Scandinavian Journal of Immunology* 33(3):319-327, 1991.

12. Gupta S, Vayuvegula B. A comprehensive immunological analysis in chronic fatigue syndrome. *Scandinavian Journal of Immunology* 33(3):319-327, 1991.

13. Morrison LJ, Behan WH, Behan PO. Changes in natural killer cell phenotype in patients with post-viral fatigue syndrome. *Clinical and Experimental Immunology* 83:441-446, 1991.

14. DuBois E. Gamma globulin therapy for chronic mononucleosis syndrome. *AIDS Research and Human Retroviruses* 2(1):S191-S195, 1986.

15. Kibler R, Lucas DO, Hicks M et al. Immune function in chronic active Epstein-Barr virus infection. *Journal of Clinical Immunology* 5:46-54, 1985.

16. Ojo-Amaise EA, Conley EJ, Peters JB. Decreased natural killer cell activity is associated with severity of chronic fatigue immune deficiency syndrome. *Clinical Infectious Diseases* 18:S157-S159, 1994.

17. See D, Broumand N, Sahl L, Tilles JG. In vitro effect of echinacea and ginseng on natural killer and antibody-dependent cell cytotoxicity in healthy subjects and chronic fatigue syndrome or acquired immunodeficiency syndrome. *Immunopharmacology* 35:229-235, 1997.

18. Straus SE, Tosato G, Armstrong G et al. Persisting illness and fatigue in adults with evidence of Epstein-Barr virus infection. *Annals of Internal Medicine* 102:7-16, 1985.

19. Whiteside TL, Friberg D. Natural killer cells and natural killer cell activity in chronic fatigue syndrome. *American Journal of Medicine* 1998; 105(3A): 27S-34S, 1998.

20. Levine PH, Whiteside TL, Friberg D, Bryant J, Colclough G, Herberman RB. Dysfunction of natural killer activity in a family with chronic fatigue syndrome. *Clinical Immunology & Immunopathology* 88(1):96-104 1998.

21. Gold D, Bowden R, Sixbey J et al. Chronic fatigue. A prospective clinical and virologic study. *JAMA* 264:48-53, 1990.

22. Mawle AC, Nisenbaum R, Dobbins JG, Gary HE Jr, Stewart JA, Reyes M, Steele L, Schmid DS, Reeves WC. Immune responses associated with chronic fatigue syndrome: A case-control study. *The Journal of Infectious Diseases* 175(1): 136-141, 1997.

23. Buchwald D, Komaroff AL. Review of laboratory findings for patients with chronic fatigue syndrome. *Reviews of Infectious Diseases* 13(1):S12-S18, 1991.

24. Altman C, Larratt K, Golubjatnikov R et al. Immunologic markers in the chronic fatigue syndrome. *Clinical Research* 36:845A, 1988.

25. Morte S, Castilla A, Civeira M-P, Serrano M, Prieto J. Gamma-interferon and chronic fatigue syndrome. *Lancet* 2:623-624, 1988.

26. Visser J, Blauw B, Hinloopen B, Brommer E, de Kloet ER, Kluft C, Nagelkerken L. CD4 T lymphocytes from patients with chronic fatigue syndrome have decreased interferon-gamma production and increased sensitivity to dexamethasone. *The Journal of Infectious Diseases* 177(2):451-454, 1998.

27. Morag A, Tobi M, Ravid Z et al. Increased (2'-5')-oligo-a synthetase activity in patients with prolonged illness associated with serological evidence of persistent Epstein-Barr virus infection. *Lancet* 1:744, 1982.

28. Lusso P, Salahuddin SZ, Ablashi DV et al. Diverse tropism of HBLV (human herpesvirus 6). *Lancet* 2(8561):743, 1987.

29. Borysiewicz LK, Haworth SJ, Cohen J et al. Epstein-Barr virus-specific immune defects in patients with persistent symptoms following infectious mononucleosis. *Quarterly Journal of Medicine* 58:111-121, 1986.

30. Glaser R, Kiecolt-Glaser JK. Stress-associated immune modulation: Relevance to viral infections and chronic fatigue syndrome. *American Journal of Medicine* 105(3A):35S-42S, 1998.

31. Ogawa M, Nishiura T, Yoshimura M, Horikawa Y, Yoshida H, Okajima Y, Matsumura I, Ishikawa J, Nakao H, Tomiyama Y, Kanayama Y, Kanakura Y, Matsuzawa Y. Decreased nitric oxide-mediated natural killer cell activation in chronic fatigue syndrome. *European Journal of Clinical Investigation* 28(11):937-943, 1998.

32. See D, Cimoch P, Chou S, Chang J, Tilles J. The in vitro immunodulatory effects of glyconutrients on peripheral blood mononuclear cells of patients with chronic fatigue syndrome. *Integrative Physiological & Behavioral Science* 33(3):280-287, 1998.

33. See DM, Tilles JG. Alpha-interferon treatment of patients with chronic fatigue syndrome. *Immunological Investigations* 25(1-2):153-164, 1996.

Neopterin

1. Bagasra O, Fitzharis JW, Bagasra TT. Neopterin: an early marker of development of pre-AIDS conditions in HIV-seropositive individuals. *Clinical Immunology Newsletter* 9:197-199, 1988.

2. Fuchs D, Muur C, Reibnegger G, Weiss G, Werner ER, Werner-Felmayer G, Wachter H. Nitric oxide synthase and antimicrobial armature of human macrophages. *The Journal of Infectious Diseases* 169:224, 1994.

3. Fuchs D, Baier-Bitterlich G, Wachter H. Nitric oxide and AIDS dementia. *New England Journal of Medicine* 333(8):521-522, 1995.

4. Baier-Bitterlich G, Fuchs D, Murr C, Reibnegger G, Werner Felmayer G, Sgonc R, Böck G, Dierich MP, Wachter H. Effect of neopterin and 7,8-dihydroneopterin on tumor necrosis factor-alpha induced programmed cell death. *FEBS Letters* 364:234-238, 1995.

5. Buchwald D, Wener MH, Pearlman T, Kith P. Markers of inflammation and immune activation in chronic fatigue and chronic fatigue syndrome. *The Journal of Rheumatology* 24(2):372-6, 1997.

6. Chao CC, Gallagher M, Phair J, Peterson PK. Serum neopterin and interleukin-6 levels in chronic fatigue syndrome. *The Journal of Infectious Diseases* 162:1412-1413, 1990.

7. Chao CC, Janoff EN, Hu S, Thomas K, Gallagher M, Tsang M, Peterson PK. Altered cytokine release in peripheral blood mononuclear cell cultures from patients with the chronic fatigue syndrome. *Cytokine* 3:292-298, 1991.

8. Linde A, Andersson B, Svenson SB, Ahrne H, Carlsson M, Forsberg P, Hugo H, Karstop A, Lenkei R, Lindwall A et al. Serum levels of lymphokines and soluble cellular receptors in primary EBV infection and in patients with chronic fatigue syndrome. *The Journal of Infectious Diseases* 165:994-1000, 1992.

9. Patarca R, Lugtendorf S, Antoni M, Klimas NG, Fletcher MA. Dysregulated expression of tumor necrosis factor in the chronic fatigue immune dysfunction syndrome: Interrelations with cellular sources and patterns of soluble immune mediator expression. *Clinical Infectious Diseases* 18:S147-S153, 1994.

10. Lutgendorf S, Klimas NG, Antoni M, Brickman A, Fletcher MA. Relationships of cognitive difficulties to immune measures, depression and illness burden in chronic fatigue syndrome. *Journal of Chronic Fatigue Syndrome* 1(2):23-41, 1995.

11. Patarca R, Klimas NG, Garcia MN, Pons H, Fletcher MA. Dysregulated expression of soluble immune mediator receptors in a subset of patients with chronic fatigue syndrome: Categorization of patients by immune status. *Journal of Chronic Fatigue Syndrome* 1:79-94, 1995.

12. Patarca R. Pteridines and neuroimmune function and pathology. *Journal of Chronic Fatigue Syndrome* 3(1):69-86, 1997.

13. Fuchs D, Moller AA, Reibnegger G et al. Decreased serum tryptophan in patients with HIV-1 infection correlates with increased serum neopterin and with neurologic/psychiatric symptoms. *Journal of AIDS* 3:873-876, 1990.

14. Iwagaki H, Hizuta A, Tanaka N, Orita K. Decreased serum tryptophan in patients with cancer cachexia correlates with increased serum neopterin. *Immunological Investigations* 24(3):467-478, 1995.

15. Heyes MP, Saito K, Milstein S, Schiff SJ. Quinolinic acid in tumors, hemorrhage and bacterial infections of the central nervous system in children. *Journal of Neurological Science* 133(1-2):112-118, 1995.

16. Saito K. Biochemical studies on AIDS dementia complex—possible contribution of quinolinic acid during brain damage. *Rinsho Byori-Japanese Journal of Clinical Pathology* 43(9):891-901, 1995.

17. Shaskan EG, Brew BJ, Rosenblum M, Thompson RM, Price RW. Increased neopterin levels in brains of patients with human immunodeficiency virus type 1 infection. *Journal of Neurochemistry* 59(4):1541-1546, 1992.

18. Andondonskaja-Renz B, Zeitler H. Pteridines in plasma and in cells of peripheral blood tumor patients. *Biochemical and Clinical Aspects of Pteridines,* Pfeiderer W, Wachter H, Curtius HC (eds.), Berlin-New York, Walter de Gruyter, 1984, pp 295-311.

19. Sonnerborg A, Saaf J, Alexius B et al. Quantitative detection of brain aberrations in human immunodeficiency virus type 1-infected individuals by magnetic resonance imaging. *The Journal of Infectious Diseases* 162:1245-1251, 1990.

20. Buchwald D, Cheney PR, Peterson DL, Henry B et al. Chronic illness characterized by fatigue, neurologic and immunologic disorders and active human herpesvirus 6 type infection. *Annals of Internal Medicine* 116:103-113, 1992.

Neuroendocrinology

1. Demitrack MA. Neuroendocrine correlates of chronic fatigue syndrome: A brief review. *Journal of Psychiatric Research* 31(1):69-82, 1997.

2. Demitrack MA. Neuroendocrine aspects of chronic fatigue syndrome: A commentary. *American Journal of Medicine* 105(3A):11S-14S, 1998.

3. Poteliakhoff A. Fatigue syndromes and the aetiology of autoimmune disease. *Journal of Chronic Fatigue Syndrome* 4(4):31-50, 1998.

4. Jones TH, Wadler S, Hupart KH. Endocrine-mediated mechanisms of fatigue during treatment with interferon-alpha. *Seminars in Oncology* 25(1 Suppl 1):54-63, 1998.

5. Baschetti R. Similarity of symptoms in chronic fatigue syndrome and Addison's disease. *European Journal of Clinical Investigation* 27(12):1061-1062, 1997.

6. Sterzl I, Zamrazil V. Endocrinopathy in the differential diagnosis of chronic fatigue syndrome, *Vnitrni Lekarstvi* 42(9):624-626, 1996.

7. Anisman H, Baines MG, Berczi I, Bernstein CN, Blennerhassett MG, Gorczynski RM, Greenberg AH, Kisil FT, Mathison RD, Nagy E, Nance DM, Perdue MH, Pomerantz DK, Sabbadini ER, Stanisz A, Warrington RJ. Neuroimmune mechanisms in health and disease: 2. Disease. *CMAJ* 155(8):1075-1082, 1996.

8. Korszun A, Papadopoulos E, Demitrack M, Engleberg C, Crofford L. The relationship between temporomandibular disorders and stress-associated syndromes. *Oral Surgery, Oral Medicine, Oral Pathology, Oral Radiology, & Endodontics* 86(4):416-20, 1998.

9. Baschetti R. High androgen levels in chronic fatigue patients. *Journal of Clinical Endocrinology & Metabolism* 81(7):2752-2753, 1996.

10. Scott LV, Dinan TG. Urinary cortisol excretion in chronic fatigue syndrome, major depression and in health volunteers. *Journal of Affective Disorders* 47(1-3):49-54, 1998.

11. Strickland P, Morriss R, Wearden A, Deakin B. A comparison of salivary cortisol in chronic fatigue syndrome, community depression and healthy controls. *Journal of Affective Disorders* 47(1-3):191-194, 1998.

12. Demitrack MA, Crofford LJ. Evidence for and pathophysiologic implications of hypothalamic-pituitary-adrenal axis dysregulation in fibromyalgia and chronic fatigue syndrome. *Annals of the New York Academy of Science* 840: 684-697, 1998.

13. Scott LV, Medbak S, Dinan TG. Blunted adrenocorticotropin and cortisol responses to corticotropin-releasing hormone stimulation in chronic fatigue syndrome. *Acta Psychiatrica Scandinavica* 97(6):450-457, 1998.

14. Scott LV, Medbak S, Dinan TG. The low dose ACTH test in chronic fatigue syndrome and in health. *Clinical Endocrinology* 48(6):733-737, 1998.

15. Scott LV, Burnett F, Medbak S, Dinan TG. Naloxone-mediated activation of the hypothalamic-pituitary-adrenal axis in chronic fatigue syndrome. *Psychological Medicine* 28(2):285-293, 1998.

16. MacHale SM, Cavanagh JT, Bennie J, Carroll S, Goodwin GM, Lawrie SM. Diurnal variation of adrenocortical activity in chronic fatigue syndrome. *Neuropsychobiology* 38(4):213-217, 1998.

17. Young AH, Sharpe M, Clements A, Dowling B, Hawton KE, Cowen PJ. Basal activity of the hypothalamic-pituitary-adrenal axis in patients with the chronic fatigue syndrome (naurasthenia). *Biological Psychiatry* 43(3):236-237, 1998.

18. Wood B, Wessely S, Papadopoulos A, Poon L, Checkley S. Salivary cortisol profiles in chronic fatigue syndrome. *Neuropsychobiology* 37(1):1-4, 1998.

19. Sharpe M, Hawton K, Clements A, Cowen PJ. Increased brain serotonin function in men with chronic fatigue syndrome. *British Medical Journal* 315(7101):164-165, 1997.

20. Dinan TG, Majeed T, Lavelle E, Scott LV, Berti C, Behan P. Blunted serotonin-mediated activation of the hypothalamic-pituitary-adrenal axis in chronic fatigue syndrome. *Psychoneuroendocrinology* 22(4):261-267, 1997.

21. Bennett AL, Mayes DM, Fagioli LR, Guerriero R, Komaroff AL. Somtomedin C (insulin-like growth factor I) levels in patients with chronic fatigue syndrome. *Journal of Psychiatric Research* 31(1):91-96, 1997.

22. Buchwald D, Umali J, Stene M. Insulin-like growth factor-I (somatomedin C) levels in chronic fatigue syndrome and fibromyalgia. *The Journal of Rheumatology* 23(4):739-742, 1996.

23. Berwaerts J, Moorkens G, Abs R. Review of neuroendocrine disturbances in the chronic fatigue syndrome: Indications for a role of the growth hormone-IGF-1 axis in the pathogenesis. *Journal of Chronic Fatigue Syndrome* 4(4):81-92, 1998.

24. Allain TJ, Bearn JA, Coskeran P, Jones J, Checkley A, Butler J, Wessely S, Miell JP. Changes in growth hormone, insulin, insulin-like growth factors (IGFs), and IGF-binding protein-1 in chronic fatigue syndrome. *Biological Psychiatry* 41(5):567-573, 1997.

25. Vara-Thorbeck R, Guerrero JA, Ruiz-Requena E, Garcia-Carriazo M. Can the use of growth hormone reduce the postoperative fatigue syndrome? *World Journal of Surgery* 20(1):81-6; discussion 86-7, 1996.

26. Cannon JG, Angel JB, Abad LW, O'Grady J, Lundgren N, Fagioli L, Komaroff AL. Hormonal influences on stress-induced neutrophil mobilization in health and chronic fatigue syndrome. *Journal of Clinical Immunology* 18(4): 291-298, 1998.

27. Visser J, Blauw B, Hinloopen B, Brommer E, de Kloet ER, Kluft C, Nagelkerken L. CD4 T lymphocytes from patients with chronic fatigue syndrome have decreased interferon-gamma production and increased sensitivity to dexamethasone. *The Journal of Infectious Diseases* 177(2):451-454, 1998.

28. Bruno RL, Creange SJ, Frick NM. Parallels between post-polio fatigue and chronic fatigue syndrome: A common pathophysiology? *American Journal of Medicine* 105(3A):66S-73S, 1998.

29. Sharpe M, Clements A, Hawton K, Young AH, Sargent P, Cowen PJ. Increased prolactin response to buspirone in chronic fatigue syndrome. *Journal of Affective Disorders* 41(1):71-76, 1996.

30. McKenzie R, O'Fallon A, Dale J, Demitrack M, Sharma G, Deloria M, Garcia-Borreguero D, Blackwelder W, Straus SE. Low dose hyrdrocortisone for treatment of chronic fatigue syndrome: A randomized controlled trial. *JAMA* 280(12): 1061-1066, 1998.

Neurofeedback treatment

1. James LC, Folen RA. EEG biofeedback as a treatment for chronic fatigue syndrome: A controlled case report. *Behavioral Medicine* 22(2):77-81, 1996.

Neuroimaging

1. Lange G, Wang S, DeLuca J, Natelson BH. Neuroimaging in chronic fatigue syndrome. *American Journal of Medicine* 105(3A):50S-53S, 1998.

2. Gonzalez MB, Cousins JC, Doraiswamy PM. Neurobiology of chronic fatigue syndrome. *Progress in Neuro-Psychopharmacology & Biological Psychiatry* 20(5):749-759, 1996.

3. Fischler B, D'Haenen H, Cluydts R, Michiels V, Demets K, Bossuyt A, Kaufman L, De Meirleir K. Comparison of 99m TcHMPAO SPECT scan between chronic fatigue syndrome, major depression and healthy controls: An exploratory study of clinical correlates of regional cerebral blood flow. *Neuropsychobiology* 34(4):175-183, 1996.

4. Fischler B, Flamen P, Everaert H, Bossuyt A, De Meirleir K. Physiopathological significance of 99mTc HMPAO SPECT scan anomalies in chronic fatigue syndrome. *Journal of Chronic Fatigue Syndrome* 4(4):15-30, 1998.

5. Greco A, Tannock C, Brostoff J, Costa DC. Brain MR in chronic fatigue syndrome. *American Journal of Neuroradiology* 18(7):1265-1269, 1997.

6. Richardson J, Campos Costa D. Relationship between SPECT scans and buspirone tests in patients with ME/CFS. *Journal of Chronic Fatigue Syndrome* 4(3):23-38, 1998.

7. Roelcke U, Kappos L, Lechner-Scott J, Brunnschweiler H, Huber S, Ammann W, Plohmann A, Dellas S, Maguire RP, Missimer J, Radu EW, Steck A, Leenders KL. Reduced glucose metabolism in the frontal cortex and basal ganglia of multiple sclerosis patients with fatigue: A 18F-flurodeoxyglucose positron emission tomography study. *Neurology* 48(6):1566-1571, 1997.

8. Tirelli U, Chierichetti F, Tavio M, Simonelli C, Bianchin G, Zanco P, Ferlin G. Brain positron emission tomography (PET) in chronic fatigue syndrome: Preliminary data. *American Journal of Medicine* 105(3A):54S-58S, 1998.

9. Nixon PG. Brainstem hypoperfusion in CFS. *Quarterly Journal of Medicine* 89(2):163-164, 1996.

10. Nixon PG. Brainstem perfusion in CFS. *Quarterly Journal of Medicine* 89(3):237, 1996.

Neurophysiology

1. Hilgers A, Frank J, Bolte P. Prolongation of central motor conduction time in chronic fatigue syndrome. *Journal of Chronic Fatigue Syndrome* 4(2):23-32, 1998.

2. Saggini R, Pizzigallo E, Vecchiet J, Macellari V, Giacomozzi C. Alteration of spatial-temporal parameters of gait in chronic fatigue syndrome, *Journal of Neurological Sciences* 154(1):18-25, 1998.

3. Neri G, Bianchedi M, Croce A, Moretti A. "Prolonged" decay test and auditory brainstem responses in the clinical diagnosis of the chronic fatigue syndrome. *Acta Otorhinolaryngologica Italica* 16(4):317-323, 1996.

4. Sendrowski DP, Buker EA, Gee SS. An investigation of sympathetic hypersensitivity in chronic fatigue syndrome. *Optometry & Vision Sciences* 74(8): 660-663, 1997.

Neuropsychology

1. Christodoulou C, DeLuca J, Lange G, Johnson SK, Sisto SA, Korn L, Natelson BH. Relation between neuropsychological impairment and functional disability in patients with chronic fatigue syndrome. *Journal of Neurology, Neurosurgery & Psychiatry* 64(4):431-434, 1998.

2. Wearden A, Appleby L. Cognitive performance and complaints of cognitive impairment in chronic fatigue syndrome (CFS). *Psychological Medicine* 27(1): 81-90, 1997.

3. DeLuca J, Johnson SK, Ellis SP, Natelson BH. Cognitive functioning is impaired with chronic fatigue syndrome devoid of psychiatric disease. *Journal of Neurology, Neurosurgery & Psychiatry* 62(2):151-155, 1997.

4. Wearden AJ, Appleby L. Research on cognitive complaints and cognitive functioning in patients with chronic fatigue syndrome (CFS): What conclusions can we draw? *Journal of Psychosomatic Research* 41(3):197-211, 1996.

5. Fry AM, Martin M. Cognitive idiosyncracies among children with the chronic fatigue syndrome: Anomalies in self-reported activity levels. *Journal of Psychosomatic Research* 41(3):213-223, 1996.

6. Michiels V, Cluydts R, Fischler B. Attention and verbal learning in patients with chronic fatigue syndrome. *Journal of the International Neuropsychology Society* 4(5):456-466, 1998.

7. Vercoulen JH, Bazelmans E, Swanink CM, Galama JM, Fennis JF, van der Meer JW, Bleijenberg G. Evaluating neuropsychological impairment in chronic fatigue syndrome. *Journal of Clinical & Experimental Neuropsychology* 20(2): 144-156, 1998.

8. Kane RL, Gantz NM, DiPino RK. Neuropsychological and psychological functioning in chronic fatigue syndrome. *Neuropsychiatry, Neuropsychology, & Behavioral Neurology* 10(1):25-31, 1997.

9. Fairhurst D, Waterman M, Lynch S. Cognitive slowing in chronic fatigue syndrome. *Psychosomatic Medicine* 59(6):638, 1997.

10. Tiersky LA, Johnson SK, Lange G, Natelson BH, DeLuca J. Neuropsychology of chronic fatigue syndrome: A critical review. *Journal of Clinical & Experimental Neuropsychology* 19(4):560-586, 1997.

11. Servatius RJ, Tapp WN, Bergen MT, Pollet CA, Drastal SD, Tiersky LA, Desai P, Natelson BH. Impaired associative learning in chronic fatigue syndrome. *Neuroreport* 9(6):1153-1157, 1998.

12. Marshall PS, Forstot M, Callies A, Peterson PK, Schenck CH. Cognitive slowing and working memory difficulties in chronic fatigue syndrome. *Psychosomatic Medicine* 59(1):58-66, 1997.

13. Marshall PS, Watson D, Steinberg P, Cornblatt B, Peterson PK, Callies A, Schenck CH. An assessment of cognitive function and mood in chronic fatigue syndrome. *Biological Psychiatry* 39(3):199-206, 1996.

14. Lakein DA, Fantie BD, Grafman J, Ross S, O'Fallon A, Dale J, Straus SE. Patients with chronic fatigue syndrome and accurate feeling-of-knowing judgments. *Journal of Clinical Psychology* 53(7):635-645, 1997.

15. Vollmer-Conna U, Wakefield D, Lloyd A, Hickie I, Lemon J, Bird KD, Westbrook RF. Cognitive deficits in patients suffering from chronic fatigue syndrome, acute infective illness or depression. *British Journal of Psychiatry* 171: 377-381, 1997.

16. DiPino RK, Kane RL. Neurocognitive functioning in chronic fatigue syndrome. *Neuropsychology Review* 6(1):47-60, 1996.

17. Michiels V, Cluydts R, Fischler B, Hoffmann G, Le Bon O, De Meirleir K. Cognitive functioning in patients with chronic fatigue syndrome. *Journal of Clinical & Experimental Neuropsychology* 18(5):666-677, 1996.

18. Johnson SK, DeLuca J, Diamond BJ, Natelson BH. Selective impairment of auditory processing in chronic fatigue syndrome: A comparison with multiple sclerosis and healthy controls. *Perceptual & Motor Skills* 83(1):51-62, 1996.

19. LaManca JJ, Sisto SA, DeLuca J, Johnson SK, Lange G, Pareja J, Cook S, Natelson BH. Influence of exhaustive treadmill exercise on cognitive functioning in chronic fatigue syndrome. *American Journal of Medicine* 105(3A):59S-65S, 1998.

20. Blackwood SK, MacHale SM, Power MJ, Goodwin GM, Lawrie SM. Effects of exercise on cognitive and motor function in chronic fatigue syndrome and depression. *Journal of Neurology, Neurosurgery & Psychiatry* 65(4):541-546, 1998.

21. Joyce E, Blumenthal S, Wessely S. Memory, attention, and executive function in chronic fatigue syndrome. *Journal of Neurology, Neurosurgery & Psychiatry* 60(5):495-503, 1996.

22. Marcel B, Komaroff AL, Fagioli LR, Kornish RJ II, Albert MS. Cognitive deficits in patients with chronic fatigue syndrome. *Biological Psychiatry* 40(6): 535-541, 1996.

23. Findley JC, Kerns R, Weinberg LD, Rosenberg R. Self-efficacy as a psychological moderator of chronic fatigue syndrome. *Journal of Behavioral Medicine* 21(4):351-362, 1998.

Neutrophils

1. Cannon JG, Angel JB, Abad LW, O'Grady J, Lundgren N, Fagioli L, Komaroff AL. Hormonal influences on stress-induced neutrophil mobilization in health and chronic fatigue syndrome. *Journal of Clinical Immunology* 18(4): 291-298, 1998.

Nutrition

1. Grant JE, Veldee MS, Buchwald D. Analysis of dietary intake and select nutrient concentrations in patients with chronic fatigue syndrome. *Journal of the American Dietetic Association* 96(4):383-386, 1996.

2. Cunliffe A, Obeid OA, Powell-Tuck J. Post-pandrial changes in measures of fatigue: Effect of a mixed or a pure carbohydrate or pure fat meal. *European Journal of Clinical Nutrition* 51(12):831-838, 1997.

3. Cunliffe A, Obeid OA, Powell-Tuck J. A placebo-controlled investigation of the effects of tryptophan or placebo on subjective and objective measures of fatigue. *European Journal of Clinical Nutrition* 52(6):425-430, 1998.

4. Bianchi GP, Grossi G, Bargossi AM. May peripheral and central fatigue be correlated? Can we monitor them by means of clinical laboratory tools? *Journal of Sports Medicine & Physical Fitness* 37(3):194-199, 1997.

5. Tanaka H, West KA, Duncan GE, Bassett DR Jr. Changes in plasma tryptophan/branched amino acid ratio in responses to training volume variation. *International Journal of Sports Medicine* 18(4):270-275, 1997.

6. Yamamoto T, Castell LM, Botella J, Powell H, Hall GM, Young A, Newsholme EA. Changes in the albumin binding of tryptophan during postoperative recovery: A possible link with central fatigue? *Brain Research Bulletin* 43(1):43-46, 1997.

7. Struder HK, Hollmann W, Platen P, Donike M, Gotzmann A, Weber K. Influence of paroxetine, branched-chain amino acids and tyrosine on neuroendocrine system responses and fatigue in humans. *Hormone & Metabolic Research* 30(4): 188-194, 1998.

8. Gastmann UA, Lehmann MJ. Overtraining and the BCAA hypothesis. *Medicine & Science in Sports & Exercise* 30(7):1173-1178, 1998.

9. Newsholme EA, Blomstrand E. The plasma level of some amino acids and mental fatigue. *Experientia* 52(5):413-415, 1996.

10. Rowbottom D, Keast D, Pervan Z, Goodman C, Bhagat C, Kakulas B, Morton A. The role of glutamine in the aetiology of the chronic fatigue syndrome: A prospective study. *Journal of Chronic Fatigue Syndrome* 4(2):3-22, 1998.

11. Haub MD, Potteiger JA, Nau KL, Webster MJ, Zebas CJ. Acute L-glutamine ingestion does not improve maximal effort exercise. *Journal of Sports Medicine & Physical Fitness* 38(3):240-244, 1998.

12. Aaserud R, Gramvik P, Olsen SR, Jensen J. Creatine supplementation delays onset of fatigue during repeated bouts of sprint running. *Scandinavian Journal of Medicine & Science in Sports* 8(5 Pt 1):247-251, 1998.

13. Greenhaff PL. Creatine supplementation: Recent developments. *British Journal of Sports Medicine* 30(4):276-277, 1996.

14. Snyder AC. Overtraining and glycogen depletion hypothesis. *Medicine & Science in Sports & Exercise* 30(7):1146-1150, 1998.

15. See DM, Cimoch P, Chou S, Chang S, Tilles J. The in vitro immunomodulatory effects of glyconutrients on peripheral blood mononuclear cells of patients with chronic fatigue syndrome. *Integrative Physiology & Behavioral Science* 33(3): 280-287, 1998.

16. Kodama M, Kodama T, Murakami M. The value of the dehydroepiandrosterone-annexed vitamin C infusion treatment in the clinical control of chronic fatigue syndrome (CFS): I. A pilot study of the new vitamin C infusion treatment with a volunteer CFS patient. *In Vivo* 10(6):575-584, 1996.

17. Kodama M, Kodama T, Murakami M. The value of the dehydroepiandrosterone-annexed vitamin C infusion treatment in the clinical control of chronic fatigue syndrome (CFS): II. Characterization of CFS patients with special reference to their response to a new vitamin C infusion treatment. *In Vivo* 10(6):585-596, 1996.

18. Wiebe E. N of 1 trials. Managing patients with chronic fatigue syndrome: Two case reports. *Canadian Family Physician* 42:2214-2217, 1996.

19. Jacobson W, Saich LK, Borysiewicz LK, Behan WMH, Behan PO, Weghitt TG. Serum folate and chronic fatigue syndrome. *Neurology* 43:2645-2647, 1993.

20. Harmon DL, McMaster D, McCluskey DR, Shields D, Whitehead AS. A common genetic variant affecting folate metabolism is not over-represented in chronic fatigue syndrome. *Annals of Clinical Biochemistry* 34 (Pt 4):427-429, 1997.

21. Kaslow JE, Ruckner L, Onishi R. Liver extract-folic acid-cyanocobalamin vs. placebo for chronic fatigue syndrome. *Archives of Internal Medicine* 149: 2501-2503, 1989.

22. Burnet RB, Yeap BB, Chatterton BE, Gaffney RD. Chronic fatigue syndrome: Is total body potassium important? *Medical Journal of Australia* 164(6): 384, 1996.

23. Tanabe K, Yamamoto A, Suzuki N, Osada N, Yokoyama Y, Samejima H, Seki A, Oya M, Murabayashi T, Nakayama M, Yamamoto M, Omiya K, Itoh H. Efficacy of oral magnesium administration on decreased exercise tolerance in a

state of chronic sleep deprivation. *Japanese Circulation Journal* 62(5):341-346, 1998.

24. Moorkens G, Keenoy M, Vertommen B, Meludu JS, Noe M, De Leeuw I. Magnesium deficit in a sample of the Belgian population presenting with chronic fatigue. *Magnesium Research* 10(4):329-337, 1997.

25. Seelig M. Review and hypothesis: Might patients with the chronic fatigue syndrome have latent tetany of magnesium deficiency? *Journal of Chronic Fatigue Syndrome* 4(2):77-108, 1998.

26. Laylander JA. A nutrient/toxin interaction theory of the etiology and pathogenesis of chronic pain-fatigue syndromes: Part I. *Journal of Chronic Fatigue Syndrome* 5(1):67-92, 1999.

27. Laylander JA. A nutrient/toxin interaction theory of the etiology and pathogenesis of chronic pain-fatigue syndromes: Part II. *Journal of Chronic Fatigue Syndrome* 5(1):93-126, 1999.

Occupational medicine

1. Mounstephen A, Sharpe M. Chronic fatigue syndrome and occupational health. *Occupational Medicine* 47(4):217-227, 1997.

2. Leese G, Chattington P, Fraser W, Vora J, Edwards R, Williams G. Short-term night shift working mimics the pituitary-adrenocortical dysfunction in chronic fatigue syndrome. *Journal of Clinical Endocrinology & Metabolism* 81(5): 1867-1870, 1996.

3. Elbers AR, Blaauw PJ, de Vries M, van Gulick PJ, Smithuis OL, Gerrits RP, Tielen MJ. Veterinary practice and occupational health. An epidemiological study of several professional groups of Dutch veterinarians: I. General physical examination and prevalence of allergy, lung function disorders and bronchial hyperreactivity. *Veterinary Quarterly* 18(4):127-131, 1996.

4. Wagner LI, Jason LA. Outcomes of occupational stressors on nurses: Chronic fatigue syndrome-related symptoms. *Nursingconnections* 10(3):41-49, 1997.

Overtraining

1. Budgett R. Fatigue and underperfomance in athletes: The overtraining syndrome. *British Journal of Sports Medicine* 32(2):107-110, 1998.

2. Hawley JA, Reilly T. Fatigue revisited. *Journal of Sports Sciences* 15(3):245-246, 1997.

3. Lehmann M, Foster C, Dickhuth HH, Gastmann U. Autonomic imbalance hypothesis and overtraining syndrome. *Medicine & Science in Sports & Exercise* 30(7):1140-1145, 1998.

4. Gabriel HH, Urhausen A, Valet G, Heidelbach U, Kindermann W. Overtraining and immune system: A prospective longitudinal study in endurance athletes. *Medicine & Science in Sports & Exercise* 30(7):1151-1157, 1998.

5. Derman W, Schwellnus MP, Lambert MI, Emms M, Sinclair-Smith C, Kirby P, Noakes TD. The "worn-out athlete": A clinical approach to chronic fatigue in athletes. *Journal of Sports Sciences* 15(3):341-351, 1997.

6. Cohen SA. Olympic fatigue syndrome. *Journal of the Medical Association of Georgia* 86(1):57-58, 1997.

Pain

1. Schmaling KB, Hamilos DL, DiClementi JD, Jones JF. Pain perception in chronic fatigue syndrome. *Journal of Chronic Fatigue Syndrome* 4(3): 13-22, 1998.

Parvovirus B19

1. Jacobson SK, Daly JS, Thorne GM, McIntosh K. Chronic parvovirus B19 infection resulting in chronic fatigue syndrome: Case history and review. *Clinical Infectious Diseases* 24(6):1048-1051, 1997.

Pediatric chronic fatigue syndrome

1. Bell DS, Robinson MZ, Pollard J, Robinson T, Floyd B. *A Parent's Guide to CFIDS.* The Haworth Medical Press, New York, 1999, pp. 1 ff.

2. de Jong LW, Prins JB, Fiselier TJ, Weemaes CM, Meijer-van den Bergh EM, Bleijenberg G. Chronic fatigue syndrome in young persons. *Nederlands Tijdschrift voor Geneeskunde* 141(31):1513-1516, 1997.

3. Jacobs G. Chronic fatigue syndrome in children. Patients organizations are denied a voice. *British Medical Journal* 315(7113):949, 1997.

4. Dowsett EG, Colby J. Chronic fatigue syndrome in children. Journal was wrong to criticize study in children. *British Medical Journal* 315(7113):949, 1997.

5. Hume M. Chronic fatigue syndrome in children. All studies must be subjected to rigorous scrutiny. *British Medical Journal* 315(7113):949, 1997.

6. Cohen P. School and the ME generation. *Nursing Times* 93(49):19, 1997.

7. Plioplys AV. Chronic fatigue syndrome should not be diagnosed in children. *Pediatrics* 100(2 Pt 1):270-271, 1997.

8. Marcovitch H. Managing chronic fatigue syndrome in children. *British Medical Journal* 314(7095):1635-1636, 1997.

9. Carter BD, Kronenberger WG, Edwards JF, Michalczyk L, Marshall GS. Differential diagnosis of chronic fatigue in children: Behavioral and emotional dimensions. *Journal of Developmental & Behavioral Pediatrics* 17(1):16-21, 1996.

10. Stein MT, First LR, Friedman SB. Twelve-year-old girl with chronic fatigue, school absence, and fluctuating somatic symptoms. *Journal of Developmental & Behavioral Pediatrics* 19(3):196-201, 1998.

11. Gibbons R, Pheby DFH, Richards C, Bray FI. Severe CFS/ME of juvenile onset—A report from the CHROME database. *Journal of Chronic Fatigue Syndrome* 4(4):67-80, 1998.

12. Arzomand ML. Chronic fatigue syndrome among school children and their special educational needs. *Journal of Chronic Fatigue Syndrome* 4(3):59-70, 1998.

13. Wright JB, Beverley DW. Chronic fatigue syndrome. *Archives of Disease in Childhood* 79(4):368-374, 1998.

14. Krilov LR, Fisher M, Friedman SB, Reitman D, Mandel FS. Course and outcome of chronic fatigue in children and adolescents. *Pediatrics* 102(2 Pt 1): 360-366, 1998.

15. Jordan KM, Landis DA, Downey MC, Osterman SL, Thurm AE, Jason LA. Chronic fatigue syndrome in children and adolescents. *Journal of Adolescent Health* 22(1):4-18, 1998.

Personality traits

1. Magnusson AE, Nias DK, White PD. Is perfectionism associated with fatigue? *Journal of Psychosomatic Research* 41(4):377-383, 1996.

2. Albus C. Chronic fatigue syndrome—A disease entity or an unspecific psychosomatic disorder? *Zeitschrift Fur Arztliche Fortbildung Und Qualitatssicherung* 91(8):717-721, 1997.

3. Johnson SK, DeLuca J, Natelson BH. Personality dimensions in the chronic fatigue syndrome: A comparison with multiple sclerosis and depression. *Journal of Psychiatric Research* 30(1):9-20, 1996.

4. Saltzstein BJ, Wyshak G, Hubbuch JT, Perry JC. A naturalistic study of the chronic fatigue syndrome among women in primary care. *General Hospital Psychiatry* 20(5):307-316, 1998.

Phosphate

1. De Lorenzo F, Hargreaves J, Kakkar VV. Phosphate diabetes in patients with chronic fatigue syndrome. *Postgraduate Medicine Journal* 74(870):229-232, 1998.

Physical activity

1. Vercoulen JH, Bazelmans E, Swanink CM, Fennis JF, Galama JM, Jongen PJ, Hommes O, Van der Meer JW, Bleijenberg G. Physical activity in chronic fatigue syndrome: Assessment and its role in fatigue. *Journal of Psychiatric Research* 31(6):661-673, 1997.

2. Ng AV, Kent-Braun JA. Quantitation of lower physical activity in persons with multiple sclerosis. *Medicine & Science in Sports & Exercise* 29(4):517-523, 1997.

3. Lawrie SM, MacHale SM, Power MJ, Goodwin GM. Is the chronic fatigue syndrome best understood as a primary disturbance of the sense of effort? *Psychological Medicine* 27(5):995-999, 1997.

4. Jason LA, Tryon WW, Frankenberry E, King C. Chronic fatigue syndrome: Relationships of self-ratings and actigraphy. *Psychological Reports* 81(3 Pt 2): 1223-1226, 1997.

Platelet volume

1. Roberts TK, McGregor NR, Dunstan RH, Donohoe M, Murdoch RN, Hope D, Zhang S, Butt HL, Watkins JA, Taylor WG. Immunological and haematological

parameters in patients with chronic fatigue syndrome. *Journal of Chronic Fatigue Syndrome* 4(4):51-66, 1998.

Polio vaccination

1. Vedhara K, Llewelyn MB, Fox JD, Jones M, Jones R, Clements GB, Wang EC, Smith AP, Borysiewicz LK. Consequences of live poliovirus vaccine administration in chronic fatigue syndrome. *Journal of Neuroimmunology* 75(1-2):183-195, 1997.

Post-dialysis fatigue

1. Dreisbach AW, Hendrickson T, Beezhold D, Riesenberg LA, Sklar AH. Elevated levels of tumor necrosis factor-alpha in post-dialysis fatigue. *International Journal of Artificial Organs* 21(2):83-86, 1998.
2. Patarca R, Perez G, Gonzalez A, Garcia-Morales RO, Gamble R, Klimas NG, Fletcher MA. Comprehensive evaluation of acute immunological changes induced by cuprophane and polysulfone membranes in a patient on chronic hemodialysis. *American Journal of Nephrology* 12:274-278, 1992.

Post-Lyme disease syndrome (PLS)

1. Ellenbogen C. Lyme disease. Shift the paradigm. *Archives of Family Medicine* 6(2):191-195, 1997.
2. Bujak DI, Weinstein A, Dornbush RL. Lyme disease. Clinical and neurocognitive features of the post-Lyme syndrome. *The Journal of Rheumatology* 23(8): 1392-1397, 1996.
3. Ravdin LD, Hilton E, Primeau M, Clements C, Barr WB. Memory functioning in Lyme borreliosis. *Journal of Clinical Psychiatry* 57(7):282-286, 1996.
4. Diamantis I. A case from practice (343). Chronic fatigue syndrome following Lyme borreliosis. *Schweizerische Rundschau fur Medizin Praxis* 85(9):287-288, 1996.
5. Gaudino EA, Coyle PK, Krupp LB. Post-Lyme syndrome and chronic fatigue syndrome. Neuropsychiatric similarities and differences. *Archives of Neurology* 54(11):1372-1376, 1997.

Post-polio syndrome

1. Bruno RL, Creange SJ, Frick NM. Parallels between post-polio fatigue and chronic fatigue syndrome: A common pathophysiology? *American Journal of Medicine* 105(3A):66S-73S, 1998.
2. Nollet F, Ivanyi B, de Visser M, de Jong BA. Post-polio syndrome; the limit of neuromuscular adaptation? *Nederlands Tijdschrift voor Geneeskunde* 140(22): 1169-1173, 1996.

3. Thorsteinsson G. Management of post-polio syndrome. *Mayo Clinic Proceedings* 72(7):627-638, 1997.

4. Bruno RL, Zimmerman JR, Creange SJ, Lewis T, Molzen T, Frick NM. Bromocriptine in the treatment of post-polio fatigue: A pilot study with implications for the pathophysiology of fatigue. *American Journal of Physical Medicine & Rehabilitation* 75(5):340-347, 1996.

5. Bruno RL. Abnormal movements in sleep as a post-polio sequelae. *American Journal of Physical Medicine & Rehabilitation* 77(4):339-343, 1998.

6. Bruno RL, Creange S, Zimmerman JR, Frick NM. Elevated plasma prolactin and EEG slow wave power in post-polio fatigue: Implications for a dopamine deficiency underlying post-viral fatigue syndromes. *Journal of Chronic Fatigue Syndrome* 4(2):61-76, 1998.

7. Schanke AK. Psychological distress, social support and coping behaviour among polio survivors: A 5-year perspective in 63 polio patients. *Disability & Rehabilitation* 19(3):108-116, 1997.

Post–Q-fever fatigue syndrome

1. Ayres JG, Flint N, Smith EG, Tunnicliffe WS, Fletcher TJ, Hammond K, Ward D, Marmion BP. Post-infection fatigue syndrome following Q fever. *Quarterly Journal of Medicine* 91(2):105-123, 1998.

2. Bennett BK, Hickie IB, Vollmer-Conna US, Quigley B, Brennan CM, Wakefield D, Douglas MP, Hansen GR, Tahmindjis AJ, Lloyd AR. The relationship between fatigue, psychological and immunological variables in acute infectious illness. *Australian & New Zealand Journal of Psychiatry* 32(2):180-186, 1998.

3. Penttila IA, Harris RJ, Storm P, Haynes D, Worswick DA, Marmion BP. Cytokine dysregulation in the post–Q-fever fatigue syndrome. *Quarterly Journal of Medicine* 91(8):549-560, 1998.

Prognosis

1. Fukuda K, Dobbins JG, Wilson LJ, Dunn RA, Wilcox K, Smallwood D. An epidemiologic study of fatigue with relevance for the chronic fatigue syndrome. *Journal of Psychiatric Research* 31(1):19-29, 1997.

2. Joyce J, Hotopf M, Wessely S. The prognosis of chronic fatigue and chronic fatigue syndrome: A systematic review. *Quarterly Journal of Medicine* 90(3): 223-33, 1997.

3. Vercoulen JH, Swanink CM, Fennis JF, Galama JM, van der Meer JW, Bleijenberg G. Prognosis in chronic fatigue syndrome: A prospective study on the natural course. *Journal of Neurology, Neurosurgery & Psychiatry* 60(5):489-494, 1996.

4. Aylward M. Government's expert group has reached a consensus on prognosis of chronic fatigue syndrome. *British Medical Journal* 313(7061):885, 1996.

Psychiatric morbidity

1. Russo J, Katon W, Clark M, Kith P, Sintay M, Buchwald D. Longitudinal changes associated with improvement in chronic fatigue patients. *Journal of Psychosomatic Research* 45(1 Spec No):67-76, 1998.

2. Morriss RK, Wearden AJ. Screening instruments for psychiatric morbidity in chronic fatigue syndrome. *Journal of the Royal Society of Medicine* 91(7): 365-368, 1998.

3. Jain SS, DeLisa JA. Chronic fatigue syndrome: A literature review from a psychiatric perspective. *American Journal of Physical Medicine & Rehabilitation* 77(2):160-167, 1998.

4. Buchwald D, Pearlman T, Kith P, Katon W, Schmaling K. Screening for psychiatric disorders in chronic fatigue and chronic fatigue syndrome. *Journal of Psychosomatic Research* 42(1):87-94, 1997.

5. Farmer A, Chubb H, Jones I, Hillier J, Smith A, Borysiewicz L. Screening for psychiatric morbidity in subjects presenting with chronic fatigue syndrome. *British Journal of Psychiatry* 168(3):354-358, 1996.

6. Krupp LB, Pollina D. Neuroimmune and neuropsychiatric aspects of chronic fatigue syndrome. *Advances in Neuroimmunology* 6(2):155-167, 1996.

7. Fischler B, Cluydts R, De Gucht Y, Kaufman L, De Meirleir K. Generalized anxiety disorder in chronic fatigue syndrome. *Acta Psychiatrica Scandinavica* 95(5):405-413, 1997.

8. Griffiths RA, Beumont PJ, Moore GM, Touyz SW. Chronic fatigue syndrome and dieting disorders: Diagnosis and management problems. *Australian & New Zealand Journal of Psychiatry* 30(6):834-838, 1996.

9. Hotopf M, Noah M, Wessely S. Chronic fatigue and minor psychiatric morbidity after viral meningitis: A controlled study. *Journal of Neurology, Neurosurgery & Psychiatry* 60(5):504-549, 1996.

Psychoneuroimmunology

1. Solomon GF. Psychoneuroimmunology and chronic fatigue syndrome: Toward new models of disease. *Journal of Chronic Fatigue Syndrome* 1(1):3-7, 1995.

2. Shanks N, Francis D, Zalcman S, Meaney MJ, Anisman H. Alterations in central cathecolamines associated with immune responses in adult and aged mice. *Brain Research* 666(1):77-87, 1994.

3. Besedovsky H, del Rey A, Sorkien E, Da Prada M, Burri R, Honegger C. The immune response evokes changes in brain noradrenergic neurons. *Science* 221(4610):564-566, 1983.

4. Vasina IG, Frolov EP, Serebriakov NG. Sympathico-adrenal system activity in a primary immune response. *Zhurnal Mikrobiologii, Epidemiologii i Imunobiologii* 10(9):88-92, 1975.

5. Boranic M. The central nervous system and immunity. *Lijecnicki Vjesnik* 112(9-10):329-334, 1990.

6. Boranic M, Pericic D, Radacic M, Poljak-Blasi M, Sverko V, Miljenovic G. Immunological and neuroendocrine responses of rats to prolonged or repeated stress. *Biomedicine & Pharmacotherapy* 36(1):23-28, 1982.

7. Basso AM, Depiante-Depaoli M, Molina VA. Chronic variable stress facilitates tumoral growth: reversal by imipramine administration. *Life Sciences* 50(23): 1789-1796, 1992.

8. Foley FW, Traugott U, LaRocca NG, Smith CR, Perlman KR, Caruso LS, Scheinberg LC. A prospective study of depression and immune dysregulation in multiple sclerosis. *Archives of Neurology* 49(3):238-244, 1992.

9. De Souza EB. Corticotropin-releasing factor and interleukin-1 receptors in the brain-endocrine-immune axis. Role in stress response and infection. *Annals of the New York Academy of Sciences* 697:9-27, 1993.

10. Irwin M. Stress-induced immune suppression. Role of the autonomic nervous system. *Annals of the New York Academy of Sciences* 697:203-218, 1993.

11. Weiss JM, Quan N, Sundar SK. Widespread activation and consequences of interleukin-1 in the brain. *Annals of the New York Academy of Sciences* 741: 338-357, 1994.

12. Herbert TB, Cohen S. Depression and immunity: a meta-analytic review. *Psychology Bulletin* 113:472-486, 1993.

13. Irwin M, Patterson T, Smith TL, Caldwell C, Brown SA, Gillin JC, Grant I. Reduction of immune function in life stress and depression. *Biological Psychiatry* 27:222-230, 1990.

14. Irwin M, Caldwell C, Smith TL, Brown S, Schuckit MA, Gillin C. Major depressive disorder, alcoholism, and reduced natural killer cell cytotoxicity. *Archives of General Psychiatry* 47:713-719, 1990.

15. Schleifer SJ, Keller SE, Bond RN, Cohen J, Stein M. Major depressive disorder: role of age, sex, severity and hospitalization. *Archives of General Psychiatry* 46:81-87, 1989.

16. Lechin F, van der Dijs B, Acosta E, Gomez F, Lechin E, Arocha L. Distal colon motility and clinical parameters in depression. *Journal of Affective Disorders* 5:19-26, 1983.

17. Lechin F, van der Dijs B, Gomez F, Arocha L, Acosta E, Lechin E. Distal colon motility as a predictor of antidepressant response to fenfluramine, imipramine and clomipramine. *Journal of Affective Disorders* 5:27-35, 1983.

18. Lechin F, van der Dijs B, Jakubowicz D et al. Effects of clonidine on blood pressure, noradrenaline, cortisol, growth hormone and prolactin plasma levels in low and high intestinal tone depressed patients. *Neuroendocrinology* 41:156-162, 1985.

19. Lechin F, van der Dijs B, Jakubowicz D et al. Role of stress in the exacerbation of chronic illness: Effects of clonidine administration on blood pressure and plasma norepinephrine, cortisol, growth hormone and prolactin concentrations. *Psychoneuroendocrinology* 12:117-129, 1987.

20. Lechin F, van der Dijs B, Amat J, Lechin M. Central neuronal pathways involved in depressive syndrome: Experimental findings. *Neurochemistry and Clini-*

cal Disorders: Circuitry of Some Psychiatric and Psychosomatic Syndromes. Lechin F, van der Dijs B (eds.), Boca Raton, FL, CRC press, 1989, pp 65-89.

21. Lechin F, van der Dijs B, Lechin A et al. Plasma neurotransmitters and cortisol in chronic illness: Role of stress. *Journal of Medicine* 25:181-192, 1994.

Psychopathology

1. Robbins JM, Kirmayer LJ, Hemami S. Latent variable models of functional somatic distress. *Journal of Nervous & Mental Disease* 185(10):606-615, 1997.

2. Wessely S. Chronic fatigue syndrome: A 20th century illness? *Scandinavian Journal of Work, Environment & Health* 23 (Suppl 3):17-34, 1997.

3. Cheung F, Lin KM. Neurasthenia, depression and somatoform disorder in a Chinese-Vietnamese woman migrant. *Culture, Medicine & Psychiatry* 21(2): 247-258, 1997.

4. Simpson M. A body with chronic fatigue syndrome as a battleground for the fight to separate from the mother. *Journal of Analytical Psychology* 42(2):201-216, 1997.

5. Holland P. Coniunctio—in bodily and psychic modes: Dissociation, devitalization and integration in a case of chronic fatigue syndrome. *Journal of Analytical Psychology* 42(2):217-236, 1997.

6. Bennett A. A view of the violence contained in chronic fatigue syndrome. *Journal of Analytical Psychology* 42(2):237-251, 1997.

7. Chagpar A. Chronic fatigue syndrome: A prodrome to psychosis? *Canadian Journal of Psychiatry—Revue Canadienne de Psychiatrie* 41(8):536-537, 1996.

8. Wessely S, Chalder T, Hirsch S, Wallace P, Wright D. Psychological symptoms, somatic symptoms, and psychiatric disorder in chronic fatigue and chronic fatigue syndrome. *American Journal of Psychiatry* 153(8):1050-1059, 1996.

9. Fischler B, Dendale P, Michiels V, Cluydts R, Kaufman L, De Meirleir K. Physical fatigability and exercise capacity in chronic fatigue syndrome: Association with disability, somatization and psychopathology. *Journal of Psychosomatic Research* 42(4):369-78, 1997.

10. Johnson SK, DeLuca J, Natelson BH. Assessing somatization disorder in the chronic fatigue syndrome. *Psychosomatic Medicine* 58(1):50-57, 1996.

11. Fischler B, Cluydts R, De Gucht Y, Kaufman L, De Meirleir K. Generalized anxiety disorder in chronic fatigue syndrome. *Acta Psychiatrica Scandinavica* 95(5):405-413, 1997.

12. de Portugal Alvarez J, Rivera Berrio L, Gonzalez San Martin F, Sanchez Rodriguez A, de Portugal E, del Rivero F. Etiology of isolated general malaise. *Anales de Medicina Interna* 13(10):471-5, 1996.

13. Johnson SK, DeLuca J, Natelson BH. Depression in fatiguing illness: Comparing patients with chronic fatigue syndrome, multiple sclerosis and depression. *Journal of Affective Disorders* 39(1):21-30, 1996.

14. Moss-Morris R, Petrie KJ, Large RG, Kydd RR. Neuropsychological deficits in chronic fatigue syndrome: Artifact or reality? *Journal of Neurology, Neurosurgery & Psychiatry* 60(5):474-477, 1996.

15. Vollmer-Conna U, Wakefield D, Lloyd A, Hickie I, Lemon J, Bird KD, Westbrook RF. Cognitive deficits in patients suffering from chronic fatigue syndrome, acute infective illness or depression. *British Journal of Psychiatry* 171:377-381, 1997.

16. Morehouse RL, Flanigan M, MacDonald DD, Braha D, Shapiro C. Depression and short REM latency in subjects with chronic fatigue syndrome. *Psychosomatic Medicine* 60(3):347-351, 1998.

17. Gruber AJ, Hudson JI, Pope HG Jr. The management of treatment-resistant depression in disorders on the interface of psychiatry and medicine. Fibromyalgia, chronic fatigue syndrome, migraine, irritable bowel syndrome, atypical facial pain, and premenstrual dysphoric disorder. *Psychiatric Clinics of North America* 19(2):351-369, 1996.

18. White PD, Cleary KJ. An open study of the efficacy and adverse effects of moclobemide in patients with the chronic fatigue syndrome. *International Clinical Psychopharmacology* 12(1):47-52, 1997.

Psychosocial measures

1. Barsky AJ, Borus JF. Functional somatic syndromes. *Annals of Internal Medicine* 130:910-921, 1999.

2. Goodwin SS. The marital relationship and health in women with chronic fatigue and immune dysfunction syndrome: Views of wives and husbands. *Nursing Research* 46(3):138-46, 1997.

3. Cope H, Mann A, Pelosi A, David A. Psychosocial risk factors for chronic fatigue and chronic fatigue syndrome following presumed viral illness: A case-control study. *Psychological Medicine* 26(6):1197-1209, 1996.

4. Ware NC. Sociosomatics and illness in chronic fatigue syndrome. *Psychosomatic Medicine* 60(4):394-401, 1998.

5. Brooks P, McFarlane AC, Newman S, Rasker JJ. Psychosocial measures. *The Journal of Rheumatology* 24(5):1008-1011, 1997.

Quality of life (QOL)

1. Anderson JS, Ferrans CE. The quality of life of persons with chronic fatigue syndrome. *Journal of Nervous & Mental Disease* 185(6):359-367, 1997.

2. Manu P, Affleck G, Tennen H, Morse PA, Escobar JI. Hypochondriasis influences quality of life outcomes in patients with chronic fatigue. *Psychotherapy & Psychosomatics* 65(2):76-81, 1996.

Red blood cell distribution width

1. Roberts TK, McGregor NR, Dunstan RH, Donohoe M, Murdoch RN, Hope D, Zhang S, Butt HL, Watkins JA, Taylor WG. Immunological and haematological parameters in patients with chronic fatigue syndrome. *Journal of Chronic Fatigue Syndrome* 4(4):51-66, 1998.

Regulation of respiration

1. Bazelmans E, Bleijenberg G, Vercoulen JH, van der Meer JW, Folgering H. The chronic fatigue syndrome and hyperventilation. *Journal of Psychosomatic Research* 43(4):371-377, 1997.
2. Lavietes MH, Bergen MT, Natelson BH. Measurement of CO_2 in chronic fatigue syndrome patients. *Journal of Chronic Fatigue Syndrome* 4(3):3-12, 1998.
3. Baschetti R. Lung function test findings in patients with chronic fatigue syndrome (CFS). *Australian & New Zealand Journal of Medicine* 27(3):346, 1997.
4. De Lorenzo F, Hargreaves J, Kakkar VV. Lung function in patients with chronic fatigue syndrome (CFS). *Australian & New Zealand Journal of Medicine* 26(4):563-564, 1996.

Rehabilitation

1. Essame CS, Phelan S, Aggett P, White PD. Pilot study of a multidisciplinary inpatient rehabilitation of severely incapacitated patients with the chronic fatigue syndrome. *Journal of Chronic Fatigue Syndrome* 4(2):51-60, 1998.

Rh blood group

1. Roberts TK, McGregor NR, Dunstan RH, Donohoe M, Murdoch RN, Hope D, Zhang S, Butt HL, Watkins JA, Taylor WG. Immunological and haematological parameters in patients with chronic fatigue syndrome. *Journal of Chronic Fatigue Syndrome* 4(4):51-66, 1998.

Rnase L

1. Suhadolnik RJ, Peterson DL, O'Brien K, Cheney PR, Herst CV, Reichenbach NL, Kon N, Horvath SE, Iacono KT, Adelson ME, De Meirleir K, De Becker P, Charubala R, Pfleiderer W. Biochemical evidence for a novel low molecular weight 2-5-A-dependent RNase L in chronic fatigue syndrome. *Journal of Interferon & Cytokine Research* 17(7):377-385, 1997.

Ross River virus

1. Bennett BK, Hickie IB, Vollmer-Conna US, Quigley B, Brennan CM, Wakefield D, Douglas MP, Hansen GR, Tahmindjis AJ, Lloyd AR. The relationship between fatigue, psychological and immunological variables in acute infectious illness. *Australian & New Zealand Journal of Psychiatry* 32(2):180-186, 1998.

Seasonal affective disorder

1. Terman M, Levine SM, Terman JS, Doherty S. Chronic fatigue syndrome and seasonal affective disorder: Comorbidity, diagnostic overlap, and implications for treatment. *American Journal of Medicine* 105(3A):115S-124S, 1998.

2. Garcia-Borreguero D, Dale JK, Rosenthal NE, Chiara A, O'Fallon A, Bartko JJ, Straus SE. Lack of seasonal variation of symptoms in patients with chronic fatigue syndrome. *Psychiatry Research* 77(2):71-77, 1998.

Selective serotonin reuptake inhibitors (SSRIs)

1. Cleare AJ, Wessely S. Fluoxetine and chronic fatigue syndrome. *Lancet* 347(9017):1770; discussion 1771-1772, 1996. Lynch S, Seth R. *Lancet* 347(9017): 1771; discussion 1271-1272, 1996. Sharma A, Kendall MJ, Oyebode F, Jones D. *Lancet* 347(9017):1770-1771; discussion 1771-1172, 1996.

2. Vercoulen JH, Swanink CM, Zitman FG, Vreden SG, Hoofs MP, Fennis JF, Galama JM, van der Meer JW, Bleijenberg G. Randomised, double-blind, placebo-controlled study of fluoxetine in chronic fatigue syndrome. *Lancet* 347(9005): 858-861, 1996.

3. Struder HK, Hollmann W, Platen P, Donike M, Gotzmann A, Weber K. Influence of paroxetine, branched-amino acids and tyrosine on neuroendocrine system responses and fatigue in humans. *Hormone & Metabolic Research* 30(4): 188-194, 1998.

4. Deale A, Chalder T, Wessely S. Commentary on randomised, double-blind, placebo-controlled trial of fluoxetine and graded exercise for chronic fatigue syndrome. *British Journal of Psychiatry* 172:491-492, 1998.

5. Lynch S, Fraser J. Fluoxetine and graded exercise in chronic fatigue syndrome. *British Journal of Psychiatry* 173:353, 1998.

Sick building syndrome (SBS)

1. Citterio A, Sinforiani E, Verri A, Cristina S, Gerosa E, Nappi G. Neurological symptoms of the sick building syndrome: Analysis of a questionnaire. *Functional Neurology* 13(3):225-230, 1998.

2. Mendell MJ, Fisk WJ, Deddens JA, Seavey WG, Smith AH, Smith DF, Hodgson AT, Daisey JM, Goldman LR. Elevated symptom prevalence associated with ventilation type in office buildings. *Epidemiology* 7(6):583-589, 1996.

3. Chester AC, Levine PH. The natural history of concurrent sick building syndrome and chronic fatigue syndrome. *Journal of Psychiatric Research* 31(1):51-57, 1997.

4. Maehara N, Sasaki T, Watanabe A, Sugimoto Y, Hayashi T, Eri Y, Suzumura H, Asaji K, Furuya E. Significance of measuring urinary 17-ketosteroid sulfates at the workplace. *Rinsho Byori—Japanese Journal of Clinical Pathology* 46(6): 553-559, 1998.

5. Sudakin DL. Toxigenic fungi in a water-damaged building: An intervention study. *American Journal of Industrial Medicine* 34(2):183-190, 1998.

6. Shefer A, Dobbins JG, Fukuda K, Steele L, Koo D, Nisenbaum R, Rutherford GW. Fatiguing illness among employees in three large state office buildings, California, 1933: Was there an outbreak? *Journal of Psychiatric Research* 31(1): 31-43, 1997.

Silicone breast implants

1. Levenson T, Greenberger PA, Murphy R. Peripheral blood eosinophilia, hyperimmunoglobulinemia A and fatigue: Possible complications following rupture of silicone breast implants. *Annals of Allergy, Asthma, & Immunology* 77(2): 119-122, 1996.
2. Rosenberg NL. The neuromythology of silicone breast implants. *Neurology* 46(2):308-314, 1996.

Sleep

1. Stores G, Fry A, Crawford C. Sleep abnormalities demonstrated by home polysomnography in teenagers with chronic fatigue syndrome. *Journal of Psychosomatic Research* 45(1 Spec No):85-91, 1998.
2. Morriss RK, Wearden AJ, Battersby L. The relation of sleep difficulties to fatigue, mood and disability in chronic fatigue syndrome. *Journal of Psychosomatic Research* 42(6):597-605, 1997.
3. Morehouse RL, Flanigan M, MacDonald DD, Braha D, Shapiro C. Depression and short REM latency in subjects with chronic fatigue syndrome. *Psychosomatic Medicine* 60(3):347-351, 1998.
4. Fischler B, Le Bon O, Hoffmann G, Cluydts R, Kaufman L, De Meirleir K. Sleep anomalies in the chronic fatigue syndrome: A comorbidity study. *Neuropsychobiology* 35(3):115-122, 1997.
5. Ambrogetti A, Olson LG, Sutherland DC, Malcolm JA, Bliss D, Gyulay SG. Daytime sleepiness and REM sleep abnormalities in chronic fatigue: A case series. *Journal of Chronic Fatigue Syndrome* 4(1):23-36, 1998.
6. Lichstein KL, Means MK, Noe SL, Aguillard RN. Fatigue and sleep disorders. *Behaviour Research & Therapy* 35(8):733-740, 1997.
7. Sharpley A, Clements A, Hawton K, Sharpe M. Do patients with "pure" chronic fatigue syndrome (naurasthenia) have abnormal sleep? *Psychosomatic Medicine* 59(6):592-596, 1997.

Soluble CD8 (sCD8)

1. Linde A, Andersson B, Svenson SB, Ahrne H, Carlsson M, Forsberg P, Hugo H, Karstop A, Lenkei R, Lindwall A et al. Serum levels of lymphokines and soluble cellular receptors in primary EBV infection and in patients with chronic fatigue syndrome. *The Journal of Infectious Diseases* 165:994-1000, 1992.

Soluble ICAM-1 (sICAM-1)

1. Patarca R, Klimas NG, Sandler D, Garcia MN, Fletcher MA. Interindividual immune status variation patterns in patients with chronic fatigue syndrome: associa-

tion with the tumor necrosis factor system and gender. *Journal of Chronic Fatigue Syndrome* 2(1):13-19, 1995.

2. Gupta S, Aggarwal S, See D, Starr A. Cytokine production by adherent and non-adherent mononuclear cells in chronic fatigue syndrome. *Journal of Psychiatric Research* 31(1):149-156, 1997.

Spleen

1. Miller BJ, Whiting JL, Clouston AD. Coincidental splenectomy in chronic fatigue syndrome. *Journal of Chronic Fatigue Syndrome* 4(1):37-42, 1998.

Stress

1. Glaser R, Kiecolt-Glaser JK. Stress-associated immune modulation: Relevance to viral infections and chronic fatigue syndrome. *American Journal of Medicine* 105(3A):35S-42S, 1998.

2. Beh HC. Effect of noise stress on chronic fatigue syndrome patients. *Journal of Nervous & Mental Disease* 185(1):55-58, 1997.

3. Cleare AJ, Wessely S. Chronic fatigue syndrome: A stress disorder? *British Journal of Hospital Medicine* 55(9):571-574, 1996.

4. Korszun A, Papadopoulos E, Demitrack M, Engleberg C, Crofford L. The relationship between temporomandibular disorders and stress-associated syndromes. *Oral Surgery, Oral Medicine, Oral Pathology, Oral Radiology, & Endodontics* 86(4):416-420, 1998.

Tapanui flu

1. St George IM. Did Cook's sailors have Tapanui flu?—Chronic fatigue syndrome on the resolution. *New Zealand Medical Journal* 109(1014):15-17, 1996.

Thyroxine

1. Dzurec LC. Experiences of fatigue and depression before and after low dose 1-thyroxine supplementation in essentially euthyroid individuals. *Research in Nursing & Health* 1997; 20(5):389-398, 1997.

Tumor growth factor-beta (TGF-beta)

1. Bennett AL, Chao CC, Hu S, Buchwald D, Fagioli LR, Schur PH, Peterson PK, Komaroff AL. Elevation of bioactive transforming growth factor-beta in serum from patients with chronic fatigue syndrome. *Journal of Clinical Immunology* 17(2):160-166, 1997.

Tumor necrosis factors (TNFs) and soluble TNF receptors

1. Beutler B, Cerami A. Cachectin (tumor necrosis factor). A macrophage hormone governing cellular metabolism and inflammatory response. *Endocrinological Reviews* 9:57-66, 1988.

2. Patarca R, Lugtendorf S, Antoni M, Klimas NG, Fletcher MA. Dysregulated expression of tumor necrosis factor in the chronic fatigue immune dysfunction syndrome: Interrelations with cellular sources and patterns of soluble immune mediator expression. *Clinical Infectious Diseases* 18:S147-S153, 1994.

3. Kriegler M, Perez C, DeFay et al. A novel form of TNF-cachectin in a cell surface cytotoxic transmembrane protein: ramifications for the complex physiology of TNF. *Cell* 53:45-53, 1988.

4. Gupta S, Aggarwal S, See D, Starr A. Cytokine production by adherent and non-adherent mononuclear cells in chronic fatigue syndrome. *Journal of Psychiatric Research* 31(1):149-156, 1997.

5. Patarca R, Fletcher MA, Klimas NG. Immunological correlates of the chronic fatigue syndrome. *Journal of Chronic Fatigue Syndrome,* P Goodnick, NG Klimas (eds.). Washington, American Psychiatric Press, 1992, pp. 1-21.

6. Dreisbach AW, Hendrickson T, Beezhold D, Riesenberg LA, Sklar AH. Elevated levels of tumor necrosis factor alpha in postdialysis fatigue. *International Journal of Artificial Organs* 21(2):83-86, 1998.

7. Lloyd A, Hickie I, Hickie C, Dwyer J, Wakefield D. Cell-mediated immunity in patients with chronic fatigue syndrome, healthy controls and patients with major depression. *Clinical and experimental Immunology* 87(1):76-79, 1992.

8. Rasmussen AK, Nielsen AH, Andersen V, Barington T, Bendtzen K, Hansen MB, Nielsen L, Pederson BK, Wiik A. Chronic fatigue syndrome—a controlled cross-sectional study. *The Journal of Rheumatology* 21(8):1527-1531, 1994.

9. Peakman M, Deale A, Field R, Mahalingam M, Wessely S. Clinical improvement in chronic fatigue syndrome is not associated with lymphocyte subsets of function or activation. *Clinical Immunology & Immunopathology* 82(1):83-91, 1997.

10. Patarca R, Goodkin K, Fletcher MA. Cryopreservation of peripheral blood mononuclear cells. *Manual of Clinical Laboratory Immunology,* Rose NR, de Macario EC, Folds JD, Lane HC, Nakamura RM (eds.), 1995, pp. 281-286.

11. Patarca R, Klimas NG, Garcia MN, Pons H, Fletcher MA. Dysregulated expression of soluble immune mediator receptors in a subset of patients with chronic fatigue syndrome: Categorization of patients by immune status. *Journal of Chronic Fatigue Syndrome* 1:79-94, 1995.

12. Patarca R, Klimas NG, Sandler D, Garcia MN, Fletcher MA. Interindividual immune status variation patterns in patients with chronic fatigue syndrome: association with the tumor necrosis factor system and gender. *Journal of Chronic Fatigue Syndrome* 2(1):13-19, 1995.

Urinary metabolites

1. McGregor NR, Dunstan RH, Zerbes M, Butt HL, Roberts TK, Klineberg IJ. Preliminary determination of a molecular basis of chronic fatigue syndrome. *Biochemistry & Molecular Medicine* 57(2):73-80, 1996.

2. McGregor NR, Dunstan RH, Zerbes M, Butt HL, Roberts TK, Klineberg IJ. Preliminary determination of the association between symptom expression and urinary metabolites in subjects with chronic fatigue syndrome. *Biochemistry & Molecular Medicine* 58(1):85-92, 1996.

Yersinia

1. Swanink CM, Stolk-Engelaar VM, van der Meer JW, Vercoulen JH, Bleijenberg G, Fennis, JM, Galama JM, Hoogkamp-Korstanje JA. *Yersinia enterocolitica* and the chronic fatigue syndrome. *Journal of Infection* 36(3):269-272, 1998.

Index

Order Your Own Copy of
This Important Book for Your Personal Library!

CONCISE ENCYCLOPEDIA OF CHRONIC FATIGUE SYNDROME

_____ in hardbound at $69.95 (ISBN: 0-7890-0922-6)

_____ in softbound at $24.95 (ISBN: 0-7890-0923-4)

COST OF BOOKS_____

OUTSIDE USA/CANADA/
MEXICO: ADD 20%_____

POSTAGE & HANDLING_____
(US: $3.00 for first book & $1.25
for each additional book)
Outside US: $4.75 for first book
& $1.75 for each additional book)

SUBTOTAL_____

IN CANADA: ADD 7% GST_____

STATE TAX_____
(NY, OH & MN residents, please
add appropriate local sales tax)

FINAL TOTAL_____
(If paying in Canadian funds,
convert using the current
exchange rate. UNESCO
coupons welcome.)

☐ **BILL ME LATER:** (\$5 service charge will be added)
(Bill-me option is good on US/Canada/Mexico orders only;
not good to jobbers, wholesalers, or subscription agencies.)

☐ Check here if billing address is different from
shipping address and attach purchase order and
billing address information.

Signature_____

☐ **PAYMENT ENCLOSED: $**_____

☐ **PLEASE CHARGE TO MY CREDIT CARD.**

☐ Visa   ☐ MasterCard   ☐ AmEx   ☐ Discover
☐ Diner's Club

Account # _____

Exp. Date _____

Signature _____

Prices in US dollars and subject to change without notice.

NAME _____

INSTITUTION _____

ADDRESS _____

CITY _____

STATE/ZIP _____

COUNTRY _____ COUNTY (NY residents only) _____

TEL _____ FAX _____

E-MAIL_____
May we use your e-mail address for confirmations and other types of information? ☐ Yes   ☐ No

Order From Your Local Bookstore or Directly From
The Haworth Press, Inc.
10 Alice Street, Binghamton, New York 13904-1580 • USA
TELEPHONE: 1-800-HAWORTH (1-800-429-6784) / Outside US/Canada: (607) 722-5857
FAX: 1-800-895-0582 / Outside US/Canada: (607) 772-6362
E-mail: getinfo@haworthpressinc.com
PLEASE PHOTOCOPY THIS FORM FOR YOUR PERSONAL USE.

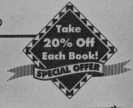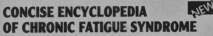
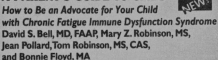